stress event
↓
perep meaningful
↓
disorg
↓
open/closer test ⟨ adap
                    method

weeks 14-27

The second trimester

weeks 28-40

The third trimester

Art editor
Christine Wood

Project assistant
Caroline Davison

Illustrators
Biz Hull
Shelagh McNicholas
Annabel Milne

Production
Mano Mylvaganam

Picture research
Abigail Ahern

This revised edition first published in 1993 by
Conran Octopus Limited
37 Shelton Street
London WC2H 9HN

Text copyright © 1988 Nina Grunfeld
Artwork copyright © 1988 Conran Octopus

The right of Nina Grunfeld to be identified as
author of this work has been asserted by her in
accordance with the Copyright, Designs and
Patents Act 1988.

This edition first published in 1995 by
Smithmark Publishers, Inc.
16 East 32nd Street
New York, NY 10016

SMITHMARK books are available for bulk
purchase sales promotion and premium use.
For details write or call the manager of special
sales, SMITHMARK Publishers Inc., 16 East 32nd
Street, New York, NY 10016; (212) 532-6600.

ISBN 0-8317-9420-8

Printed in Hong Kong

10 9 8 7 6 5 4 3 2 1

*i*NTRODUCTION

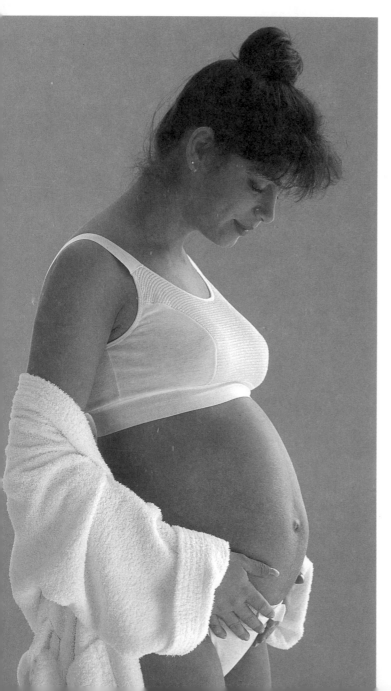

*t*his book is a week-by-week guide to what is happening to you and your baby throughout your pregnancy.

On the left-hand pages, 'You and Your Developing Baby' describes the physical and emotional changes you experience and the detailed development of your baby. You will find this a useful guideline although, of course, every woman - and every pregnancy – is different so you may feel that what appears under 'You' in Week 7, for example, fits your Week 9, or even 11, better. In the same way, the weights given for the baby can only be a guide.

You may like to use the diary space on the left-hand pages to write down important appointments and keep a note of your feelings; this will make an interesting record of your pregnancy for later on. We have given important reminders in the relevant weeks under 'Don't forget' : for example, your first prenatal visit, making a dental appointment or noting down when you first feel your baby kick.

The right-hand pages for each week feature particular aspects of pregnancy in some detail. Some of these features, for example the amniocentesis test and ultrasound scan, are particularly relevant to a certain week while others may vary and many are relevant throughout your pregnancy. Cross-references are included wherever necessary to help you find all the information you want and there is also a full index at the back of the book.

Since medically your pregnancy is dated from the first day of your last period, and not from the time of conception, you may not know you are expecting a baby until you are at least 'five weeks pregnant' – which is actually about two to three weeks after conception, and around the time of your first missed period.

The first few weeks of this book will, in effect, have already happened! You will find them interesting to read before you start following the weeks of the guide.

Throughout the diary your baby is referred to as 'he', not because of any bias but just to differentiate you, the mother, from your baby. The term 'partner' has been chosen to cover the expectant father, no matter what his status.

During pregnancy you will come across lots of new words and terms, especially medical ones. There is a short glossary of the more important of these at the back of the book. Never allow yourself to be confused by these – always ask your health-care provider what they mean if you do not understand the terms they are using.

There is also a list of useful addresses at the end of the book. Refer to the associations or groups if you would like more information about any particular topic. The forty weeks of pregnancy are conventionally divided into three terms, known medically as 'trimesters'. Many women find that, physically and emotionally, their pregnancy falls into three parts too. Forty weeks can seem a long time and you may find it helpful to have it broken down in some way. We have used colored bands to differentiate these three terms throughout the book and to help you relate the forty weeks to the actual months of your pregnancy.

A note about the author
When she was about fifteen weeks pregnant, Nina Grunfeld decided to write a book about what happens to mothers and their babies, week by week, during pregnancy. She was by then feeling well, happy and excited about her baby and wanted to convey to other pregnant women the emotional ups and downs, the pleasures and concerns of pregnancy.

In Week 40 this book was finished and her first child, Michael, was born. Nina Grunfeld now has three children. She has written nine books and is co-author of the BBC series and book *Nanny Knows Best*.

week 1

month   date

MON

TUES

WED

THURS

FRI

SAT

SUN

*n*OTES

PREGNANCY TESTS

The first, and probably most reliable, sign of your pregnancy will be a missed period. Less reliable signs will be tiredness and a more frequent need to urinate, or you may just 'feel pregnant'. To test whether or not you are pregnant, you can buy a home testing kit at a pharmacy or you can have a pregnancy test done at your doctor's or your family planning clinic.

The most common pregnancy tests work by detecting a particular hormone in your urine. There is a more concentrated amount of this pregnancy hormone in the first urine you pass in the day, so this is the best time to do the test. Follow the instructions with a kit very carefully. Some tests can confirm pregnancy within a few days of your missed period. If your test is negative then it could be that there isn't yet enough pregnancy hormone to show up in a test. If your period doesn't start, then have another test in a week's time.

Positive results from a urine test are 99 per cent reliable.

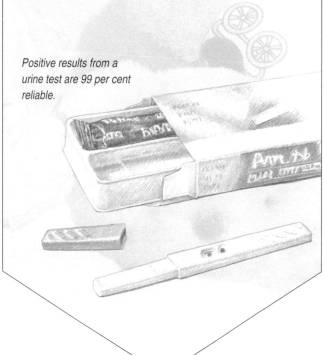

*n*OW YOU'RE PREGNANT

*C*ongratulations on your pregnancy!

You may be one of the lucky ones who find the next forty or so weeks just fly by. Or you may feel pregnancy is a long process during which your body takes over your life. Every pregnancy is different and your feelings will change over the weeks.

The first fourteen weeks of your pregnancy may well be the hardest, so if you are feeling under par in the initial stages, take heart that things will improve. Even if you've been trying to get pregnant for a long time, the reality may make you scared; pregnancy in any case tends to make you over-emotional. You may also worry about the possibility of miscarriage and about whether your baby will be all right. All these fears are perfectly normal and should be discussed with your partner and, if you wish, with your doctor or midwife.

For many women the middle term of pregnancy is the most exhilarating time of their lives. Make the most of it!

As you get more noticeably pregnant, friends will be full of advice. Listen to it all, but decide how much is relevant to you. Every woman is different and these forty weeks are a time for finding out about yourself. You may well become introspective during pregnancy. This is a good thing. Use the opportunity to rest, relax and get to know yourself. It will be the last time you have on your own for quite a while.

During pregnancy you may feel very romantic and should enjoy these feelings. Your partner no doubt will appreciate all the attention and affection and it may be some time after your baby is born before you feel so sensual again.

Towards the end of your pregnancy it is perfectly natural to feel impatient for it to be over. You may be filled with conflicting emotions: on the one hand anxious about having the child and giving birth, and yet on the other hand feeling that by now you can't wait to hold your baby. These emotions are perfectly understandable: a new member of your family is about to arrive and you are bound to feel a mixture of excitement together with a reasonable degree of nervousness.

Use this diary to write down all your thoughts and feelings over the following months. You'll enjoy rereading it in the years to come.

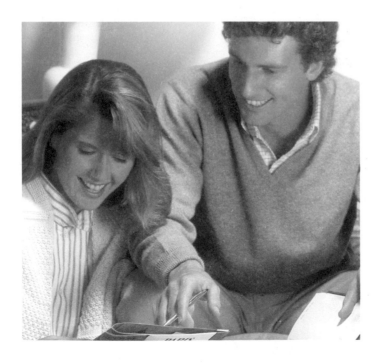

week 2

month   date

MON

TUES

WED

THURS

FRI

SAT

SUN

*n*OTES

OVULATION AND FERTILIZATION

Ovulation happens each month. It is when a ripe egg, or ovum – a single cell just 0.005in (0.13mm) large – is released from one of your ovaries and travels along your fallopian tube. At the same time the lining of your womb becomes engorged with blood ready to receive and nourish an embryo and the mucus in your cervix becomes thinner so that sperm can swim through it more easily.

Most women ovulate about fourteen days before a period, whatever the length of their menstrual cycle. For you to be pregnant, you will have had sexual intercourse shortly before or after you ovulated and your ripe egg will have been fertilized by your partner's sperm. Except in the case of twins, only one sperm will pierce the outer wall of your egg and fertilize it. Instantly the egg loses its attraction, hardens its outer shell and all the other sperm drop off.

Most of the 400 million sperm ejaculated into your vagina (1) leak out, but some swim up through your cervix, into your uterus (2) and then into your fallopian tube (3). The sperm are attracted to the ovum (4) and stick to its surface.

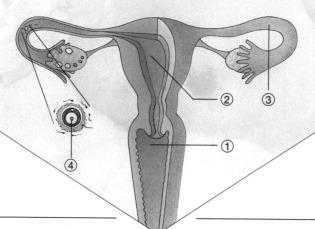

8

*P*REGNANCY DANGERS

*O*nce you know you are pregnant, it's time to become more aware of your body and learn to trust your intuition. You must consciously avoid all risks to your unborn child, which means coming to terms with the danger inherent in smoking, drinking and taking drugs. Their possible harmful effects are now known to be present throughout pregnancy not just the first trimester as is often assumed.

Smoking

It is extremely important that you stop smoking as soon as you know you are pregnant. Ask your partner to stop smoking too, passive smoking also holds dangers. If you find it impossible to give up, at least cut right down. Don't be tempted to try commercial 'patches' to help you when you are pregnant.

Smoking during pregnancy increases the risk of early miscarriage and the chances of possible complications at birth – or of a stillborn baby. It has been proved that women who smoke have a greater risk of miscarriage and tend to have smaller babies.

Pets and hygiene

Wash your hands after cleaning your cat's litter tray and after gardening (or wear gloves). Cats' feces may contain a parasite that affects many adults and children, giving mild flu symptoms. The dangers occur if this infection (toxoplasmosis) is contracted during pregnancy, when it can cause damage to the baby's brain and eyes.

Alcohol and caffeine

The safest policy is to abstain from alcohol completely, and to cut out or limit caffeine consumption during pregnancy. If you are planning to become pregnant, it is wise to cut down or stop drinking alcohol. Research shows that drinking alcohol, even in moderation, increases the risk of miscarriage or of a low-birthweight baby.

The federal Food and Drug Administration (FDA) has advised that "Pregnant women should avoid caffeine-containing foods and drugs, if possible, or consume them only sparingly."

Drugs

Don't take any drugs during pregnancy without consulting your doctor. Many drugs can cross the placenta and cause severe abnormalities in the fetus; even aspirin and sleeping tablets can be harmful, and very few antibiotics can be safely taken during the first three months of pregnancy. A few drugs do not cross the placenta and doctors are careful to prescribe only those drugs that they know to be safe.

If you suffer from any illness or disorder for which you normally take drugs, tell your doctor if you are planning to become pregnant or immediately you suspect you may be pregnant – he or she may change your course of treatment.

German measles (rubella)

If you get German measles during the first three months of pregnancy your baby may be malformed, deaf, blind or born with heart disease. Rubella can also be the cause of miscarriage or stillbirth. Check whether you have been immunized against it, and if not, keep far away from anyone who has German measles. Tell your doctor if you do come into contact with anyone who might have the disease.

HOW TO STOP SMOKING

- Think of your unborn baby, not just yourself.
- Tell everyone you are going to stop.
- Put the money you would have spent on cigarettes in a glass jar so you can see how quickly it adds up.
- Change any habits related to cigarette smoking.
- Avoid places where people are smoking.
- If you become tense, breathe deeply and practice relaxation techniques (see Week 30).

week 3

month   date

MON

TUES

WED

THURS

FRI

SAT

SUN

CONCEPTION

During the two weeks after fertilization, the cell that will become your baby multiplies quickly from a single-cell egg into over one hundred cells which will travel along your fallopian tube until they reach your uterus. It is called a blastocyst and looks like a tiny blackberry. The blastocyst is formed of two layers: the outer one eventually becomes your placenta and the inner one, your embryo.

The blastocyst floats free in the cavity of the uterus and is nurtured by 'milk' secreted from the glands in the uterus lining. By the end of Week 3 the blastocyst will begin to attach itself firmly to your specially thickened womb lining, a process known as implantation. When this has happened, conception is said to have taken place.

Implantation usually takes place in the upper part of the uterus on either the left or right side, depending on which ovary ovulated.

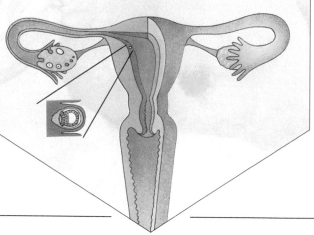

notes

bEALTHY EATING

$d$uring pregnancy remember that you are having to provide nutrition not only for yourself but also for your developing baby. This doesn't mean you should go overboard on quantity but that you should eat a good, varied, high-protein diet rich in vitamins and minerals – so start now. Eat fresh food whenever you can and try to cut out sweets, sugary drinks, cakes, canned fruit in heavy syrup, rich desserts and soups, and chocolate.

If you are hungry between meals eat raw vegetables or fresh fruit. If you follow a strict diet (vegetarian or macrobiotic), discuss this with your doctor: you may need to supplement it with extra minerals or vitamins. If you start feeling sick, follow the advice given in Week 7 and don't worry about dieting.

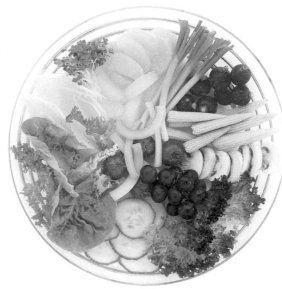

See Week 2 for Safety with Pets

See Week 19 for Vitamins and Minerals

See Week 25 for Weight gain in Pregnancy

WHAT YOU NEED IN YOUR DIET

Protein Pregnant women need at least 3oz (75g) of protein a day, especially if ill or tired. Cheese, eggs, beans and fish are good alternatives if you don't eat meat.
Carbohydrates These provide energy, but can make you fat. If you are overweight, eat whole-wheat bread and avoid foods containing sugar, alcohol, white flour and rice.
Fiber Fiber (or roughage) will help prevent constipation. Foods with high fiber content are peas and beans; whole-wheat bread and cereals; potatoes (especially their skins); fruit, vegetables and nuts.
Fats Cut down on fats. Trim fat off meat; don't fry food or drown it in rich sauces; eat low-fat yogurt and semi-skimmed milk.
Milk and dairy products Dairy products contain calcium which is important for your baby's development. Eat plenty of dairy products during pregnancy.
Vitamins and minerals (see Week 19).

SAFETY WITH FOOD

Some foods may carry infections that can cross the placenta to the baby.
● Soft cheeses such as Camembert and Brie may cause listeriosis, a rare bacterial infection. Pâté and prepared meat dishes also carry a risk.
● Avoid certain fish such as swordfish, shark and marlin which may contain dangerous levels of mercury that can harm a developing fetus. Limit your intake of tuna to one-half pound per week.
Fish contaminated with PCBs should also be avoided such as freshwater carp, wild catfish, bluefish, striped bass, and whitefish.
● Cook meat and fish well, to kill bacteria, and the parasite that causes taxoplasmosis.

week 4

month   *date*

MON

TUES

WED

THURS

FRI

SAT

SUN

*n*OTES

YOU AND YOUR DEVELOPING BABY

You This is the week of your first missed period. You may be aware of some slight body changes.

Baby During Week 4 the mass of cells embedded in your uterus multiply rapidly and group together to make different structures. The outer layer surrounding the embryo reaches out like roots sending projections into the lining of your uterus. Those which penetrate deepest form the basis of the placenta.

The inner cells of the embryo form themselves into two, then three layers, each of which will grow to be different parts of your baby's body.

Other cells are developing into the amniotic sac. By the end of the week the embryo is just visible to the naked eye.

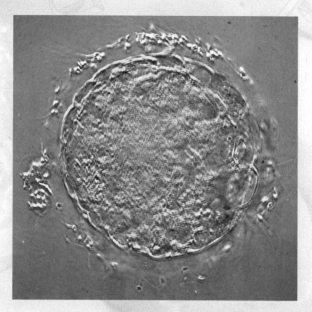

This mass of cells is an early stage of embryonic development. The surrounding pink ring is the debris of sperm that failed to penetrate the ovum.

medically your pregnancy is dated from the first day of your last period, and not from the time of conception. So, what is called 'four weeks pregnant' is actually about two weeks after conception. Worked out like this, the average pregnancy lasts for forty weeks – the length of this diary.

To work out your EDD (estimated date of delivery), you will need to know the date of your LMP (last menstrual period) and then follow this simple formula.

LMP	18.11.92
add nine months	18.08.93
add seven days	25.08.93

If your normal cycle is less than twenty eight days, your EDD may be a few days earlier, since you ovulate earlier in a short menstrual cycle; conversely, in a cycle longer than twenty-eight days you ovulate later and your EDD will be a few days after your calculated date.

Remember that this is just a rough guide – babies have a habit of arriving either early or late, hardly ever on time. Some people find it a good idea to give friends an EDD about two weeks later than the actual one as it can be quite frustrating at the end of your pregnancy being asked if the baby has arrived yet.

The trimesters

Pregnancy is divided into three trimesters (literally, thirds of pregnancy). The trimesters are a convenient way of dividing up the forty weeks of pregnancy for the medical profession, but you too will probably find that you naturally think of your pregnancy in three stages of roughly the same duration.

See Week 7 for Morning Sickness

EDD chart (right)
To find your expected date of delivery, look at the first day of your last period on the top line of figures – your EDD appears in bold type underneath.

JANUARY	1 2 3 4 5 6 7 8 9 10 11 12 13 14 15 16 17 18 19 20 21 22 23 24 25 26 27 28 29 30 31	JANUARY
OCTOBER	**8 9 10 11 12 13 14 15 16 17 18 19 20 21 22 23 24 25 26 27 28 29 30 31 1 2 3 4 5 6 7**	**NOVEMBER**
FEBRUARY	1 2 3 4 5 6 7 8 9 10 11 12 13 14 15 16 17 18 19 20 21 22 23 24 25 26 27 28	FEBRUARY
NOVEMBER	**8 9 10 11 12 13 14 15 16 17 18 19 20 21 22 23 24 25 26 27 28 29 30 1 2 3 4 5**	**DECEMBER**
MARCH	1 2 3 4 5 6 7 8 9 10 11 12 13 14 15 16 17 18 19 20 21 22 23 24 25 26 27 28 29 30 31	MARCH
DECEMBER	**6 7 8 9 10 11 12 13 14 15 16 17 18 19 20 21 22 23 24 25 26 27 28 29 30 31 1 2 3 4 5**	**JANUARY**
APRIL	1 2 3 4 5 6 7 8 9 10 11 12 13 14 15 16 17 18 19 20 21 22 23 24 25 26 27 28 29 30	APRIL
JANUARY	**6 7 8 9 10 11 12 13 14 15 16 17 18 19 20 21 22 23 24 25 26 27 28 29 30 31 1 2 3 4**	**FEBRUARY**
MAY	1 2 3 4 5 6 7 8 9 10 11 12 13 14 15 16 17 18 19 20 21 22 23 24 25 26 27 28 29 30 31	MAY
FEBRUARY	**5 6 7 8 9 10 11 12 13 14 15 16 17 18 19 20 21 22 23 24 25 26 27 28 1 2 3 4 5 6 7**	**MARCH**
JUNE	1 2 3 4 5 6 7 8 9 10 11 12 13 14 15 16 17 18 19 20 21 22 23 24 25 26 27 28 29 30	JUNE
MARCH	**8 9 10 11 12 13 14 15 16 17 18 19 20 21 22 23 24 25 26 27 28 29 30 31 1 2 3 4 5 6**	**APRIL**
JULY	1 2 3 4 5 6 7 8 9 10 11 12 13 14 15 16 17 18 19 20 21 22 23 24 25 26 27 28 29 30 31	JULY
APRIL	**7 8 9 10 11 12 13 14 15 16 17 18 19 20 21 22 23 24 25 26 27 28 29 30 1 2 3 4 5 6 7**	**MAY**
AUGUST	1 2 3 4 5 6 7 8 9 10 11 12 13 14 15 16 17 18 19 20 21 22 23 24 25 26 27 28 29 30 31	AUGUST
MAY	**8 9 10 11 12 13 14 15 16 17 18 19 20 21 22 23 24 25 26 27 28 29 30 31 1 2 3 4 5 6 7**	**JUNE**
SEPTEMBER	1 2 3 4 5 6 7 8 9 10 11 12 13 14 15 16 17 18 19 20 21 22 23 24 25 26 27 28 29 30	SEPTEMBER
JUNE	**8 9 10 11 12 13 14 15 16 17 18 19 20 21 22 23 24 25 26 27 28 29 30 1 2 3 4 5 6 7**	**JULY**
OCTOBER	1 2 3 4 5 6 7 8 9 10 11 12 13 14 15 16 17 18 19 20 21 22 23 24 25 26 27 28 29 30 31	OCTOBER
JULY	**8 9 10 11 12 13 14 15 16 17 18 19 20 21 22 23 24 25 26 27 28 29 30 31 1 2 3 4 5 6 7**	**AUGUST**
NOVEMBER	1 2 3 4 5 6 7 8 9 10 11 12 13 14 15 16 17 18 19 20 21 22 23 24 25 26 27 28 29 30	NOVEMBER
AUGUST	**8 9 10 11 12 13 14 15 16 17 18 19 20 21 22 23 24 25 26 27 28 29 30 31 1 2 3 4 5 6**	**SEPTEMBER**
DECEMBER	1 2 3 4 5 6 7 8 9 10 11 12 13 14 15 16 17 18 19 20 21 22 23 24 25 26 27 28 29 30 31	DECEMBER
SEPTEMBER	**7 8 9 10 11 12 13 14 15 16 17 18 19 20 21 22 23 24 25 26 27 28 29 30 1 2 3 4 5 6 7**	**OCTOBER**

FIRST SIGNS

Morning sickness This is a misnomer. Many women feel sick all day or just in the evenings. Some women *feel* sick, many actually are.
Tender breasts You may have already noticed your breasts becoming bigger and more sensitive as they can do before your period. They may also tingle slightly.
Tiredness You may feel faint or dizzy or exhausted: try and rest.
Food and taste Some women experience a metallic taste in their mouth which affects their sense of taste. Others just stop eating certain foods, commonly tea, coffee, alcohol, fatty and fried foods and fish. You may also get cravings for other foods.
Vaginal discharge You may notice an increase in vaginal secretions.

week 5

month   *date*

MON

TUES

WED

THURS

FRI

SAT

SUN

YOU AND YOUR DEVELOPING BABY

You The most likely sign of pregnancy is a missed period although you might mistake a little 'breakthrough bleeding', which sometimes occurs, for an ordinary period. Other early signs of pregnancy that you may experience at some stage in the next few weeks are outlined in Week 4.

Baby You baby's nervous system, spine and brain are already beginning to develop, and the cells which started off as an embryonic disc grow lengthways until your baby has a definite head and tail end.

The first stage in the development of the central nervous system is the formation of a groove in the top layer of cells towards the tail end of the embryo. The cells fold up and round to make the hollow neural tube, one end of which become your baby's brain and the other end his spinal cord. At the same time blocks of tissue begin to grow which will eventually form your baby's spine, ribs and abdominal muscles.

During Week 5 your baby is shorter than your eyelashes – about 1/10 in (2mm).

*n*OTES

*m*any women feel highly sensual during pregnancy, especially during the second trimester. Your change in libido may be due to the high level of hormones circulating in your blood. During pregnancy your sexual organs are more highly developed and many parts of your body are more sensitive and therefore more capable of arousal. Sex could also be more fun now because it can be spontaneous – there's no worry about birth control or wondering whether this will lead to a longed-for baby.

If you have had a miscarriage or difficult pregnancies in the past or are experiencing vaginal bleeding now, ask your doctor's advice about sexual intercourse during the first fourteen weeks. The only other times not to have sex are at the very end of your pregnancy, either if you have had a show (i.e. your plug of mucus is dislodged) or if your waters have broken. Otherwise sexual intercourse is safe throughout pregnancy.

See Week 1 for kits for Pregnancy Tests

See Weeks 9 and 10 for Prenatal Care

See Week 30 for Sex in Later Pregnancy

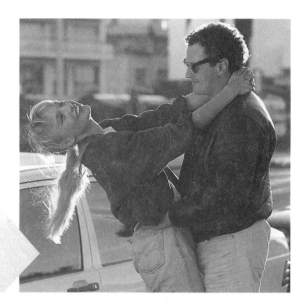

Once you know you are pregnant, you begin to realize that your relationship will soon change. During the next eight months the experiences you share will bond you together.

SEX IN PREGNANCY

Contrary to what you or your partner may believe, it is impossible for his penis, or the semen which he ejaculates, to harm your baby. The muscles of the cervix and a special plug of mucus seal off your uterus completely. Where there is a risk (see above), the miscarriage could be triggered off by your orgasm causing your uterus to contract, which might set off other contractions. But this will not happen in a normal pregnancy.

The human female is one of the very few mammals to permit sexual intercourse at any time during pregnancy so it is not surprising if sometimes you don't feel like sex. If you don't feel sexually aroused during your pregnancy, don't worry – your desire will return later. A fairly typical pattern in pregnancy is for your sex drive to decrease in the first fourteen weeks then increase again in your second trimester (Weeks 14-27); you may lose interest in sex after about Week 29, especially if you feel heavy, unattractive and uncomfortable.

week 6

month   *date*

MON

TUES

WED

THURS

FRI

SAT

SUN

YOU AND YOUR DEVELOPING BABY

You By now your uterus can be felt to be swollen and slightly enlarged – it is about the size of a tangerine. Your breasts may feel tender.

Baby Although your baby's face still can't be made out, he already has a neck, a completed rudimentary brain and a bump for a head. In the chest cavity a heart is developing.

This week the connecting stalk by which the embryo has been attached to your placenta begins to grow into the umbilical cord and blood vessels start forming within it, strengthening the link between you and your child. By the end of the week your baby has a bloodstream with a functioning circulation. Tiny limb buds appear at the corners of his body.

The lower part of the body looks more like a tail. The blocks of tissue that make up the back of the embryo develop faster than those of the front, causing him to grow in a curved shape, resembling a seahorse.

By the end of this week your baby will be ¼ in (6mm) long – the size of your little fingernail.

*n*OTES

Don't forget Make an appointment with your doctor or midwife to confirm your pregnancy.

$\mathcal{V}$ISITING THE DOCTOR

See Weeks 9 and 10 for Antenatal Care

*b*y now you will know you are pregnant, even if you haven't yet had it confirmed and you will probably be planning a visit to your doctor. If you want an out-of-the-hospital birth, you'll need to explore birthing center and/or midwifery options in your area. The National Association of Childbearing Centers provides lists of freestanding birthing centers; the American College of Nurse Midwives and the Midwives Alliance of North America can put you in touch with midwives in your area (see Useful Addresses, p. 110). Remember that no birth is ever as you expect it to be, so be prepared to change if need be.

You may not want to tell the world that you're pregnant just yet. But you must tell your doctor so that she can confirm your pregnancy and start you thinking about prenatal care.

PREPARATION

What to bring
● A list of things you wish to discuss with your doctor or midwife. Don't be embarrassed to write down the answers as you get them.
● A note to remind you of the first day of your last menstrual period, so that the date your baby is due can be worked out. Your doctor will also want to know the average length of both your periods and menstrual cycle so try and remember these.
● A sample of the first urine you passed that morning so that a pregnancy test can be done. Make sure the jar in which you bring the urine is clean and soap-free.

What to expect
● There may be variations from one obstetrician's or midwife's practice to another; from one patient to another. Some tests may be given at different visits and depending on your situation different tests may be indicated. Expect to see the doctor or midwife from now on on a monthly basis, except for the last month when you will see her every week. Expect at the first visit:
● A general physical examination (although this may be put off until the second prenatal visit).
● A detailed medical history will be taken, including your menstrual history; operations; chronic problems; medications taken regularly and in the past; drug reactions and allergies; diseases that run in the family; previous pregnancies and their outcome.
● A pelvic examination to confirm pregnancy, a Pap smear for cancer detection and vaginal exam.
● Urine tests (repeated at every visit) and blood tests (these may not start until the second or third visit). Your blood pressure will be measured at every visit.
● Discussion of vitamins, diet, activities, any special instructions.

week 7

MON

_____

TUES

_____

WED

_____

THURS

_____

FRI

_____

SAT

_____

SUN

YOU AND YOUR DEVELOPING BABY

You You may feel dizzy or faint if you stand for long periods. You may also have spells of overwhelming tiredness, which is normal. Rest as much as you can. By now you may be experiencing some of pregnancy's 'problems', including some emotional ones.

Baby The embryo is now known as a fetus. Your baby's head is beginning to assume its eventual human shape. The limb buds are growing rapidly and arms and legs starting to resemble paddle-shapes.

The ears and eyes are developing and apertures for the nostrils are appearing. Development of the jaws and mouth is continuing and the lips, tongue and first teeth buds are now visible.

By the end of this week your baby's brain and spinal cord will be almost complete. The heart now has four chambers. It is beating with enough force to circulate blood cells through the entire complex network of blood vessels.

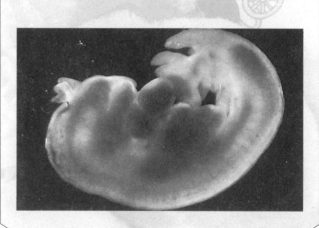

Your baby is now about the size of your thumbnail.

*n*OTES

Don't forget Start looking into prenatal classes (see Week 30) now.

mIXED EMOTIONS

You will be coming to terms with what it means to be pregnant and it is up to you when you want to tell your friends. Some women want to broadcast the news as soon as the pregnancy is confirmed, while others prefer to wait until they are sure all is well.

The first trimester may well be the worst time of your pregnancy, emotionally as well as physically. You have just taken a step into the unknown which is, let's face it, quite courageous. No matter how much you may have wanted a baby in the past, you may now be wondering if you've made the right decision. Possibly for the first time in your life, you are also being forced into a constant awareness of your body which may be making you feel sick, tired and over-emotional. You may be nervous that you are going to miscarry.

Allaying your fears

It's quite normal to worry about whether your baby is going to be all right. Thankfully only a tiny percentage of babies born today are handicapped. It is important to behave sensibly throughout your pregnancy; keep all your doctor's appointments and never be afraid to ask for medical advice on anything that is worrying you. Remember that you are asking for your baby as well as for yourself.

Most women are worried about labor. Dreams about giving birth to weird objects are common. You may find it helps to share your fears about labor with your friends or your doctor or midwife. On a broader level, you may feel worried about how the baby is going to change your life, both financially and socially. Will it end your freedom? Disrupt the happy relationship you have with your partner? You may wonder how you will cope with bringing up a child. Never let a problem get the best of you – find someone to discuss it with.

At times during your pregnancy you may have the sense of being very alone and feel that your partner isn't doing enough. You may argue more during pregnancy, but you will also feel closer. Much of this can attributed down to changing hormones. It is important to involve your partner as early as you can.

See Weeks 12 and 13 for Common Problems7

See Week 2 for Pregnancy Dangers

See Week 24 for The Father's Role

MORNING SICKNESS

By now you may have begun to feel sick. Nausea, and sometimes actual vomiting, affects about half of all pregnant women and you may feel sick at any time, day or night. The cause is thought to be related to the hormonal changes taking place in your body. Morning sickness is not serious, just very unpleasant, but with luck it will disappear by Week 14 – let your doctor know if you are still nauseous after Week 14.

If you can't keep anything down, not even drinks, tell your doctor. But otherwise, try to reduce the risk of being sick. Here are some suggestions that may help.

● Eat a cracker before getting out of bed in the morning and get up slowly.
● Eat small, light meals throughout the day.
● Drink between meals rather than with food.
● Wear clothes without waistbands.
● Put away anything that makes you feel sick, such as soaps or perfume.
● If cooking smells such as fried food make you nauseous, buy foods that don't need preparing.

week 8

MON

TUES

WED

THURS

FRI

SAT

SUN

YOU AND YOUR DEVELOPING BABY

You Your waist may be vanishing, and your breasts and nipples will be enlarging.

Baby The eyes are covered by a skin which will eventually split to form eyelids. His eyes are visible but not yet protruding. The middle part of the ear, responsible for balance as well as hearing, will have developed by the end of the week. During the next seven days he will start to open his mouth and be able to suck and chew once the upper and lower jaws fuse at the sides.

By now his heart is pumping vigorously with a regular rhythm. Blood vessels can be seen through the skin which is as thin as tracing paper. All the major internal organs are now in place although not yet fully developed.

The bones of his arms and legs are starting to harden and elongate; fingers and toes are more obvious though joined by webs of skin; and the major joints are forming.

Your baby is still smaller than your nose – 1in (2.5cm) long and fish-like in shape, with an over-large head and small body.

notes

Don't forget Make a dental appointment. Regular checkups are very important in pregnancy.

*l*OOKING GOOD

a good diet, plus plenty of rest and sleep, are extremely important throughout pregnancy. Experiment with make-up and different hairstyles if you want people to look at your face rather than your stomach. You may find you look better than ever over the next few months. The pregnancy hormones have a noticeable effect on your hair, skin and nails.

Hair Both hair and nails grow more rapidly than usual. Dry hair may become drier and greasy hair greasier. Don't experiment with perms or color just now.
Nails Nails may break or split easily. Keep them short and wear gloves for any chores. Try rubbing baby oil into the base of your nails nightly to help prevent cracking.
Breasts Don't use soap on your breasts. Buy new support bras (see below).
Skin Most women's skin improves but if yours does the opposite, don't worry – after pregnancy it will be back to normal. The extra blood circulating round your body will

make you look rosy-cheeked.
Stretch marks These may occur if the elastic fibers in your skin have become over-stretched and ruptured. Although they first appear as dramatic reddish streaks, they shrink to indistinct silvery lines afterwards. There is no sure way to avoid stretch marks. It helps not to put on too much weight.
Color changes Pigmented birthmarks and freckles can darken during pregnancy, especially if exposed to sunlight. They will lighten again after delivery. Some women may get blotchy patches on their face and neck; these are caused by pregnancy hormones. Use

make-up to cover them up if they bother you. They will start to disappear after delivery.
Teeth During pregnancy the gums around your teeth become spongier and more prone to infection – you may notice them bleeding more. Brush your teeth at least twice a day and floss them regularly. Make a dental appointment immediately and remember to avoid X-rays.
Personal hygiene You may find you sweat more, due to an increase in body weight and temperature. Wash regularly and wear cotton underwear if possible. Never douche during pregnancy.

See Week 15 for Pregnancy Wardrobe.

BUYING A BRA

Your breasts may increase as much as two bra sizes during pregnancy. Since breasts contain no muscles, they need good support if they are to return to their normal shape after childbirth. Shop where the staff are trained to fit bras. If you want to breast-feed you will need at least two nursing bras as well (see below).

Pregnancy bras These should have wide shoulder straps and adjustable fastenings to allow for later chest expansion. Make sure you buy the correct cup size. The measurement directly under your breasts is the bra size and around the fullest part of your breasts and shoulder blades indicates the cup size.

Nursing bras Usually worn both night and day so they need to be comfortable and should also have adjustable fastenings. Make sure that you can open them easily at the front with one hand – the other hand will be holding the baby. Buy them no earlier than Week 35.

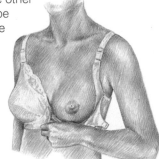

week 9

month   *date*

MON

TUES

WED

THURS

FRI

SAT

SUN

YOU AND YOUR DEVELOPING BABY

You You may begin to notice skin changes caused by pregnancy hormones. Any wrinkles may become less obvious due to your face becoming fuller. Your gums may also be thickening. Start some regular exercises; go walking or swimming every day if possible. Diving is not recommended during pregnancy.

Baby Your baby is beginning to have a more mature appearance although his head is still bent forward on his chest. The development of his eyes is now complete, although each eye still has a membrane eyelid over it. A nose has also appeared.

During Week 9 the chest cavity becomes separated from the abdominal cavity by a band of muscle that later develops into the diaphragm. The spine is making its first, tiny movements and, although you won't be able to feel it yet, your baby is starting to kick and exercise his muscles.

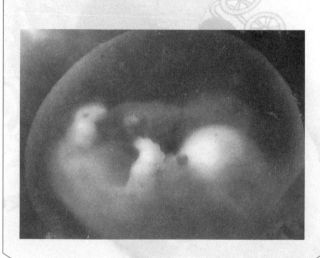

The fastest growth this week is in the limbs, hands and feet. Fingers and toes start to be defined.

$\boldsymbol{p}$RENATAL CARE/1

$\boldsymbol{n}$o matter what you may feel, or how busy you are, prenatal checkups are time well spent – for you and your baby. These routine examinations enable your doctor or widwife to detect problems that might effect your health or your child's, or influence the birth. They are also an opportunity for you to get help eliminating or controlling unhealthy habits, such as smoking cigarettes or drinking alcohol, skipping meals, and/or eating nutrition-poor foods.

Write down everything you want to discuss with your doctor or midwife before every visit – it is easy to forget things once you are there (pregnancy amnesia is famous!). If they are short of time, ask when you can come back to talk. It is important that you find the answers to everything that is worrying you. Take notes on what is said or you may forget it.

Below is a list of questions you may wish to ask. They apply mainly to hospital deliveries.

See Week 40 for The Birth

See page 88 for Understanding your Medical Records

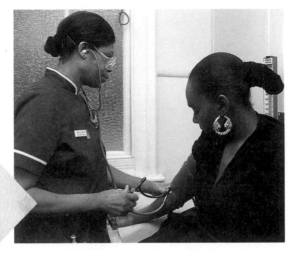

At each prenatal visit your blood pressure will be measured and a sample of urine tested. You will also be weighed and examined to check that the baby is growing satisfactorily.

(Continued in Week 10)

QUESTIONS FOR THE DOCTOR OR MIDWIFE

Prenatal care
● How often will I have prenatal appointments?
● What tests will I be given?
● Where can I go for prenatal classes? Are there other classes, such as prenatal exercise in my area?
● Will I be shown around the labor and maternity wards before the birth?

The birth
● Is my partner (or close relative or friend) welcome all the time during labor?
● What is your policy on induction, pain relief, episiotomy?
● Is an epidural available?
● Can I walk around in labor and find my own birth position?
● If I need to have a cesarean section can my partner stay with me? Can it be done with an epidural?
● If I want, will my baby be put to my breast immediately after birth?
● Is it possible to be alone with my baby and partner immediately after the birth?

The hospital
● Do you have a Special Care Nursery? If not, where is the nearest one?
● Do you have a birthing chair, a birthing pool (or other special equipment)?
● Is it possible to have my baby born in subdued lighting and a quiet atmosphere?
● What is the normal length of stay on the maternity ward?
● Are there any special rules about visiting or about numbers of visitors?
● How many beds are there to a room?
● Can the baby stay with me in my room or are babies taken to the nursery at night?

week 10

month　　　　*date*

MON

TUES

WED

THURS

FRI

SAT

SUN

*n*OTES

YOU AND YOUR DEVELOPING BABY

You Your uterus has now grown to the size of an orange. Your heart, lungs and kidneys are beginning to work harder. Your breasts will be noticeably larger and can be rather tender.

Baby Your baby's brain has developed so rapidly that his head is still large in proportion to the rest of his body. The inner part of the ears are complete and the external parts are beginning to grow.

The lungs are growing inside the chest cavity and in the abdomen, the stomach and intestine are formed and kidneys are moving into their permanent positions. The umbilical cord is properly formed and blood is circulating along it.

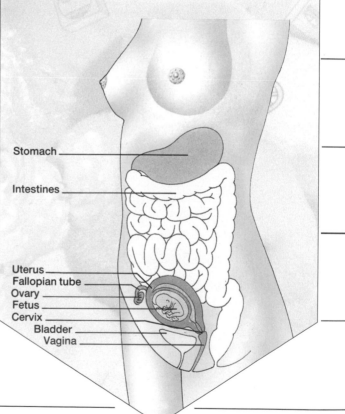

Stomach

Intestines

Uterus
Fallopian tube
Ovary
Fetus
Cervix
Bladder
Vagina

Don't forget Avoid smoke-filled rooms to protect your developing fetus.

*t*hroughout your pregnancy there will be tests and questions to make sure that you and your baby are fit and healthy. Every time you see your doctor or midwife you will be weighed, your blood pressure will be taken, your urine will be checked for protein and sugar, your uterus will be felt and, from Week 23, your baby's heartbeat will be listened to.

Your doctor will always be trying to anticipate any problems or special circumstances you may have during your pregnancy and delivery. Some of the tests are described below. Several of them are carried out on all women during pregnancy. Others are only carried out on women at risk – when an abnormality is suspected. Others, such as a test for the HIV virus, you can request if you think you may be at risk. However, many public health authorities now recommend that all pregnant women, not just those at high risk, be tested for the HIV virus.

See Week 17 for Testing in Pregnancy

ROUTINE LABORATORY TESTS

Here are the routine tests that you can expect at your prenatal visits:

Blood tests Your blood will be taken to determine your blood type and you will be given a complete blood count or CBC to see if you are anemic and need to take iron supplements. Also tests for Rh status, immunity to German measles (rubella), and syphilis.

Urine test A test for protein and sugar (glucose) in the urine done at each visit.

Hepatitus B It is now recommended for all pregnant women.

PAP tests At the initial prenatal exam and again during the postpartum exam.

Special tests Most mothers will not need any special tests at all, although they will probably have one or more sonograms or ultrasound exams as their pregnancy progresses. The tests are usually only for babies whose parents have a family history of a particular condition. They are given at different weeks and for different reasons, but they are all designed to find out if your baby has any likelihood of being born with an inherited condition or with some disability. The tests include chorionic villus sampling (see box); amniocentesis, at 15 weeks; ultrasound, which can be performed at any stage of pregnancy; blood tests and genetic counseling. MSAFP (alpha-fetoprotein) test is a blood test increasingly given to women in the second trimester; it tests for open neural tube defects and other severe problems. Genetic counseling is done before you become pregnant to guage the statistical likelihood of inherited diseases in your children.

With all these tests, the results may mean you have to take painful decisions and perhaps decide to terminate your pregnancy. Take any professional counseling you are offered and then follow your own feelings and those of your partner.

CHORIONIC VILLUS SAMPLING

This technique can take the place of amniocentesis, which is carried out so late on in the pregnancy that the mother-to-be can already feel fetal movements by the time she receives the results. C.V.S. can be performed as early as week 5 so that if any problem is detected, the decision to terminate can be made early in the pregnancy. But C.V.S. is only performed on certain women and only at a few specialized maternity hospitals. The test is painless, but there is a slight risk of suffering a miscarriage.

week 11

month   *date*

MON

TUES

WED

THURS

FRI

SAT

SUN

*n*OTES

YOU AND YOUR DEVELOPING BABY

You If you've been feeling sick during the last few weeks you may begin to feel better. Start thinking about where you want to go for prenatal classes (see Week 29).

Baby By the end of the week all your baby's essential internal organs will be formed and the majority beginning to function. From now on, these organs will simply continue to grow in size. Your baby is relatively safe from the risk of developing major congenital abnormalities.

His head is still relatively large for his body size and his limbs are still quite short and thin. His ankles and wrists have formed and his elbows and knees are taking shape. His face is beginning to look more human as it becomes more rounded. The back of the head has enlarged, so that his eyes are in a more natural position; his ears look flatter and continue to develop.

Your baby's heart is pumping blood to all parts of the body as well as through the umbilical cord to what will eventually become the placenta.

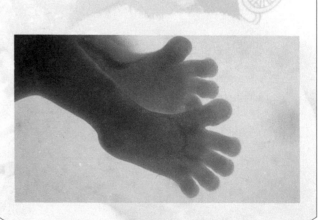

Your baby's fingers and toes are now separate and clearly developed.

Don't forget Go and see your dentist if you haven't already.

WORKING IN PREGNANCY

One positive advantage of working during pregnancy is that it takes your mind off waiting. But if your job is potentially dangerous (involving heavy lifting, contact with chemicals, lead, dangerous substances or X-rays), it is best to discuss with your doctor and employer about how safe it is to continue. If your work normally involves a lot of standing, see if you can switch to a more sedentary job for the time being. And, of course, if there is *any* medical reason why you should stop work, then do, but remember that you will need a doctor's letter. If you have any problems with your employer, try and get legal help (see below).

Sleepiness may make it impossible for you to concentrate during early pregnancy. For many this is the most difficult time in which to work. Don't push yourself – this feeling of exhaustion will only last for another few weeks. If you find yourself dropping off to sleep during the day, you need rest. Try and take some time off work until you feel less tired. Nausea may also make it hard to concentrate. Bring in food to pick at during the day.

If you have a medical complication during pregnancy and need to take more time off than your employer allows, you will need your physician's help in applying for disability benefits. Also now under the Family and Medical Leave Act, you may be able to take up to 12 weeks off, without pay. Talk with your doctor or union representative or call a hotline operated by 9 to 5 (1-800-522-0925).

See Week 7 for Morning Sickness

THE PREGNANCY DISCRIMINATION ACT
Under the Pregnancy Discrimination Act, it is illegal for a company to fire, demote or penalize a worker for being pregnant. If you suspect that you're being discriminated against, discuss your legal rights with a representative of the Equal Employment Opportunity Commission (call 800-669-4000 for the telephone of an office near you). To stay on good terms with your employer, inform her of your pregnancy at least four months before your due date so she'll have time to find a temporary or permanent replacement.

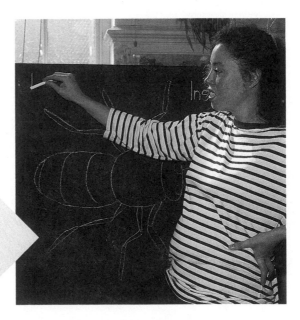

If your work involves standing for long periods of time, organize your day so that you can rest whenever possible and eat frequent snacks to keep your energy levels up.

week 12

MON

TUES

WED

THURS

FRI

SAT

SUN

*n*OTES

YOU AND YOUR DEVELOPING BABY

You Your uterus can now be felt as a hard ridge above your pubic bone. About a quarter of your pregnancy weight gain will take place from now until Week 20 (see Week 25). Most women gain 15-30lb (7-14kg) in their pregnancies. If you are underweight now, you may need to put on more than 30lb (14kg). If you are overweight, it may be a good idea to discuss a diet with your doctor to make sure you put on less than 14kg (30lb). Never start an unsupervised diet while pregnant.

Baby His brain and muscles are working so that he is kicking, curling his toes, rotating his feet and wrists, clenching and unclenching his fists, pressing his lips together, frowning and making other facial expressions. His external ears and his nails are forming.

This week the umbilical cord starts to circulate blood between the fetus and the group of membranes attached to the wall of your uterus. Your baby begins to rely on these membranes for nourishment.

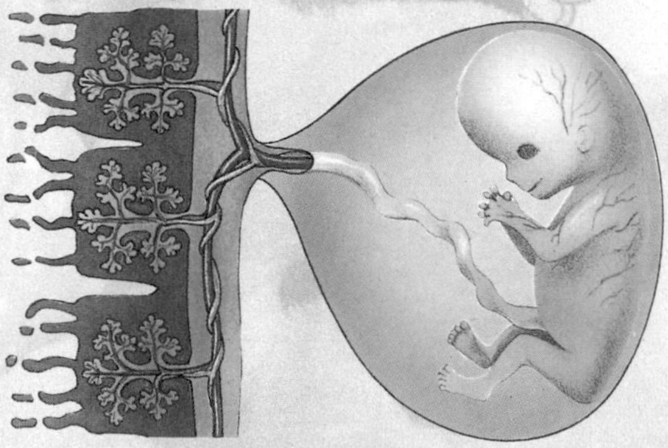

m ost of the problems mentioned here and in Week 13 are fairly common in early pregnancy and are more of a nuisance than serious. Speak to your doctor immediately, however, if you experience any of the problems highlighted in the panel.

Backache See Week 31

Bladder problems In early and late pregnancy you need to urinate more frequently. Sometimes it wakes you up at night. You could try drinking less in the evening and rocking back and forth as you urinate, which lessens the pressure on your bladder and may help empty it more completely.

Bleeding gums This can be a sign of gum infection (gingivitis). If brushing your teeth makes you nauseous, use a toothbrush with a smaller head.

Blocked nose Your nose may be more stuffed-up than usual, especially on waking up. Don't use a nasal spray or take cold cures. It will disappear after childbirth.

Constipation Drink lots of water and fruit juice and eat bran and wholewheat bread. Avoid strong laxatives and go to the bathroom the moment you feel you need to. Avoid straining as this may lead to piles.

Cramps Cramps may be due to poor blood circulation, lack of salt in the diet or low levels of calcium in the blood. It usually occurs in your legs. If it happens at night, try hopping on the foot of the affected leg or massaging it firmly for a while.

If you get a lot of cramping, go for short walks or try and stretch your calf muscles by exercising your legs in some other way before you go to bed to get the circulation going. Your doctor may give you calcium supplements.

Cystitis (bladder infection) If you have a burning feeling when urinating and you feel as if you need to urinate all the time, you may have cystitis. See your doctor immediately and drink as much water as you can.

Fainting During early and late pregnancy you may feel dizzy or unsteady and may even faint, due to the brain being relatively-deprived of blood, because your blood is rushing either to your feet (if you are standing) or to your uterus. If you feel faint, get into fresh air as soon as possible, loosen tight clothes and sit down or, if possible, lie down with your head flat and your legs raised.

Avoid standing for long periods, taking hot baths, sitting in smoky rooms and getting up quickly.

Flatulence This is due to a sluggish intestine during pregnancy. Flatulence is caused either by you swallowing air (often to stop yourself feeling sick) or eating certain foods (like beans, fried foods and onions). Avoid problem foods where possible and eat light meals.

Headaches Try not to worry if you get occasional headaches; getting plenty of rest and relaxation should help. If your headaches are frequent, with visual disturbance, tell your doctor – it may be a sign of high blood pressure.

Hemorrhoids See Piles
Incontinence See Week 26
Indigestion and heartburn See Week 26

See Week 26 for Common Problems

(Continued in Week 13)

CONTACT THE DOCTOR IF YOU

- Are vomiting excessively.
- Have any vaginal bleeding apart from around the time of your first missed period.
- Have any leak of clear fluid from your vagina.
- Fall or have an accident.
- Have swollen feet, fingers, ankles or face.
- Are short of breath.
- Have excessive dizziness or headaches.
- Have excessive white or discolored discharge.
- Have abdominal cramps.

week 13

MON

TUES

WED

THURS

FRI

SAT

SUN

YOU AND YOUR DEVELOPING BABY

You Your uterus is already swollen by your pregnancy and measures approximately 4in (10cm) in diameter. Your doctor will be able to feel it in your lower abdomen as a soft swelling coming out of your pelvis.

The main danger of miscarriage is over. From now on syphilis, rubella (German measles) and rare tropical diseases are the only known infections which can cross to the fetus and do him any harm.

You may see a dark line (the *linea nigra*) appearing down the center of your abdomen. This continues to darken during pregnancy but will fade after delivery.

Baby By the end of this week your baby is properly formed. But were he to be born, he could not survive because, although all the organs are present, they have not yet matured enough to perform the jobs for which they are intended. The rest of your pregnancy is designed to allow the fetus to grow in size, and to give his vital organs sufficient time to mature so that they are capable of independent life.

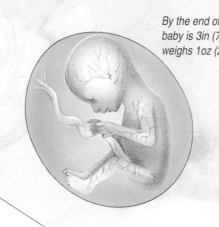

By the end of this week your baby is 3in (7.5cm) long and weighs 1oz (28g).

𝑛OTES

COMMON PROBLEMS/2

Insomnia Don't worry about not sleeping; it's more important that you relax. Try a warm milk drink at bedtime; reading a good book; having a warm bath; relaxation exercises (see Week 30). Don't take sleeping pills without advice.

Itching and skin problems
General itching – with or without a rash – can be due to poor hygiene, excess weight gain and/or sweating. Keep your body clean and apply calamine lotion or talcum powder to the affected area. Wear loose clothing made of natural fibers. Any tiny red spots, or naevi, in your skin are harmless and will disappear.

Morning sickness See Week 7

Nose bleeds During pregnancy there is an increased volume of blood in your body, including in the vessels lining your nose. Nose bleeds can easily occur if you blow your nose too hard and the vessels rupture. If your nose starts bleeding, lean forward slightly and gently apply pressure to the bridge of your nose, or pinch your nostrils together to stop the blood flow.

Piles (hemorrhoids) Piles are a form of varicose vein which occur around the anus. You may first notice some discomfort and possibly some bleeding when your bowels are opened. Piles can be caused by anything that increases pressure in your abdomen such as constipation, chronic coughing or lifting. They can be very uncomfortable, especially when defecating, and they may itch and bleed slightly especially if the pile is large and outside your rectum. Cure your constipation (see Week 12) and try to keep your stools soft and regular. Keep your anal area clean to avoid irritation and ask your doctor for creams or suppositories if necessary.

If your piles itch badly, put some crushed ice in a plastic bag, cover it with a cloth and hold the pack gently against the piles. Piles usually disappear soon after delivery.

Pins and needles See Week 26

Stretch marks See Week 8

Swelling of legs, ankles, fingers (Edema) See Week 26

Thrush Thrush is common during pregnancy and can be passed on to your baby at birth, although this can be quickly cleared up by a course of medicine. Don't wear panty hose or underpants that are too tight; ask your doctor for a prescription for creams and suppositories.

Tiredness This may go on throughout pregnancy although it often gets better in your second trimester.

Vaginal secretions An increase in vaginal secretions is normal during pregnancy due to change in vaginal tissues in preparation for the birth. If your secretions smell awful, make you sore, are painful or contain blood, tell your doctor. Otherwise, if you need to, wear a sanitary napkin (not a tampon). Never douche or use vaginal deodorant during pregnancy.

Varicose veins These can be inherited or caused by hormones or, in later pregnancy, by your enlarged womb pressing down and obstructing the flow of blood from your legs to your heart. Avoid standing or sitting still for long periods, crossing your legs, wearing tight garments or being constipated. If varicose veins do run in the family, wear support hose or stockings.

To prevent varicose veins exercise frequently, watch your weight and rest every day with legs raised above your heart. Varicose veins can also appear temporarily in the vulva where they feel like a dull ache. They too disappear after the birth.

See Week 26 for Problems of Later Pregnancy

MISCARRIAGE

It is deeply upsetting and troubling to have a miscarriage, but never feel that it is your fault – the causes of miscarriage are still largely unknown. Most miscarriages occur in the first trimester. If you have any bleeding, with or without pain, call your doctor and lie down. Your doctor will advise you how long to wait before trying to conceive again.

week 14

MON

TUES

WED

THURS

FRI

SAT

SUN

YOU AND YOUR DEVELOPING BABY

You You are beginning the middle stage of your pregnancy, generally thought of as the most enjoyable. Your uterus is now the size of a large grapefruit and you should be able to feel the top of it two fingers' breadth above your public bone.

Baby Week 14 is the beginning of the second trimester, the stage of the main growth of your baby; he increases in size, his organs mature and complex hormone and other processes develop.

Your baby has begun to grow hair: he has eyebrows and a small amount of hair on his head. His heart is beating strongly and can be heard using an ultrasonic device. His heartbeat is almost twice the rate of a normal adult's. All his major muscles are responding to stimulation from the brain. The arms can bend from the wrist and elbow, the fingers can curl, make fists and grasp: his nervous system has begun to function.

Your placenta is now fully operational; it both nourishes your fetus and produces hormones. Your child starts to drink some amniotic fluid and his kidneys begin to make a little urine which he can now pass.

Your baby now weighs 2¼ oz (65g) and measures about 4in (10cm).

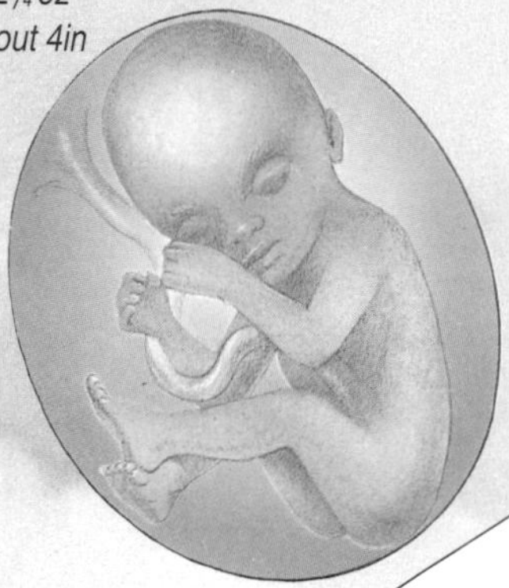

notes

32

*l*ooking after children is one of the most exhausting occupations for a pregnant woman. Learn to pick up your child with your knees bent, or kneel down to cuddle and comfort him instead of picking him up. Try not to let your attitude to your older children change.

If possible, don't talk about your pregnancy to your children too soon or they will get bored waiting. Once they know, prepare them by pointing out babies in their carriages in the street – comment on how helpless they look so that the new baby is not expected to be a playmate from the start. Show older children pictures of themselves as babies and buy them a doll of their own so they have someone to look after too. If you need a child to move out of his familiar crib, or room, do it well before the baby is born so that the two events do not appear related. Let your partner increase his involvement with your children, especially with bathing, feeding and story telling, so that you can decrease yours well before the birth.

If you are having the baby in the hospital, make arrangements for your children in advance and rehearse and discuss them frequently; it is only surprise that will worry them. When you leave for the hospital, say goodbye to them no matter what time of day or night it is. It is upsetting for children to wake up and find you gone.

If you want to have a home birth, make sure your children know what is going to happen beforehand and think about what arrangements would be best for them.

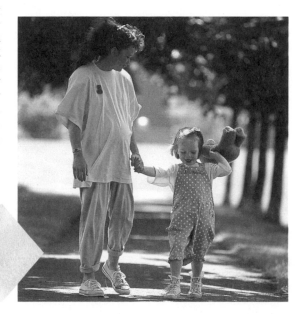

No matter how excited your child may seem about a new brother or sister, don't expect them to feel the same once the baby has arrived. It is a confusing time and children take time to adjust too. Involve them according to how much they can understand.

THE MIDDLE TERM OF PREGNANCY

Emotions The middle period of pregnancy is usually a time for feeling energetic and creative. You may begin to feel closer to other women and find yourself talking about personal things you haven't discussed before. You may love the attention from other people once they notice your belly.

The first time your baby kicks can be very exciting and may bring you much closer to him. It's the first real sign that someone separate from you is there, and that something really is happening.
Working Your excess energy can make you overdo things during your working day. No matter how strong you feel, take it easy whenever you can. Don't stand all day – this may lead to circulation problems and varicose veins later on. Put your feet up when you can. Try squatting instead of bending over which might strain your back. Always ask for help – people are happy to give it.

week 15

month   *date*

MON

TUES

WED

THURS

FRI

SAT

SUN

*n*OTES

You Your clothes are probably getting tight and you will need to wear looser garments. Your pregnancy may begin to show, though this varies from person to person. To cope with the increased amount of blood circulating in your body and your baby's need for oxygen, your enlarged heart has increased its output by twenty per cent.

Baby From now on most of your baby's energy is directed towards growing and maturing. The hair on his head is becoming thicker and he has eyelashes and eyebrows. The three tiny bones of his middle ear are the first bones to harden, which means he is probably capable of hearing, although the auditory centers in his brain, which make sense of sounds received, have not yet developed. The amniotic fluid that surrounds him is an excellent sound conductor and from now on he will hear your stomach rumbling, your heart beating and the sound of your voice. Why not sing to him?

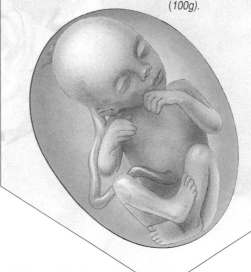

The baby now measures approximately 5¼ in (13.5cm) and weighs roughly 3½oz (100g).

SEX IN PREGNANCY

$y$ou may still be feeling nauseous and, if so, you probably would rather not have any physical contact at all – not for the present at least. But however you feel, you can be sure your emotions will change and change again as the months go by. Sooner or later your sexual relationship will be back to normal.

Even if you are lucky enough to feel like having sex during your first and second trimesters, you may find that towards the end of pregnancy you experience a loss of libido (sexual desire). It may be just that you feel heavier and more lethargic or you may feel you must be less desirable because of your changing propor-

tions. But if you both find sex exciting at this time, there is no reason why you shouldn't enjoy it. You'll probably find that the classic missionary position (with the man or woman on top) becomes uncomfortable. Try 'the spoons' position instead – you lying on your side with your partner lying close behind you, facing the same way. Or kneel or crouch so your partner can enter you from behind. Or find ways other than penetration to have sex. It's fun to massage each other. And, right at the end of your pregnancy, sex may even come in useful – they say that having orgasms may be one way of getting an overdue labor started.

See Week 5 for Your Relationship

See Week 24 for The Father's Role

PELVIC FLOOR EXERCISES

Learning to contract and release your pelvic floor muscles efficiently will help you during labor by making you supple for the birth of your baby. It will also help prevent piles, incontinence and prolapse of your uterus. To see how efficient your pelvic muscles are, the next time you urinate try to stop in mid-stream, hold for a few seconds and then relax.

You can do pelvic floor exercises lying, sitting or standing. Imagine that your pelvic floor area is a lift going up. Contract it a little until you reach the first floor. Hold it there, then take it to the second floor and so on, until your

muscles are fully contracted. Hold them for a count of six. Then release them gradually, floor by floor, until you have reached the ground floor. Now push your pelvic floor downwards or away from you, as if you were blowing a candle out with your vagina and pant with your mouth open, slowly and deeply. This is the position that your pelvic floor should be in when your baby's head is being born.

Rest and then repeat six times, making sure that you are not holding your breath, tightening your shoulders or pulling in your stomach. The rest of your body should always be totally relaxed.

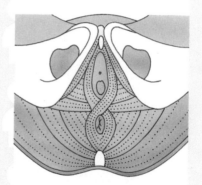

Your pelvic floor muscles are between your legs, forming a figure-8 around your front and back passages. They contract spontaneously during sexual intercouse.

week 16

month　　　　　*date*

MON

TUES

WED

THURS

FRI

SAT

SUN

*n*OTES

YOU AND YOUR DEVELOPING BABY

You You may feel the first movements of the fetus, called 'quickening', about now. It is a sort of bubbling, fluttering sensation in your stomach.

Baby He is moving vigorously although his movements are rarely felt at this stage in a first pregnancy. His head is still quite large in comparison to his body size. His face is becoming more human, although his chin is still small and his mouth wide. His eyes are enormous, closed and spaced wide apart.

A fine downy hair (lanugo) appears all over your baby's body and face which is thought to keep him at the right temperature. Most of it will disappear before birth.

The external genital organs have now developed enough for your baby's sex to be detectable by ultrasound, although your untrained eye will probably not be able to see them.

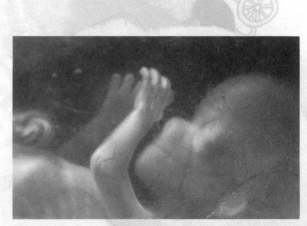

Your baby's skin is transparent, but looks red because the blood vessels can be seen through it.

Don't forget Make a note of the date when you first feel your baby move inside you.

$\mathcal{U}$ LTRASOUND

$\mathcal{U}$ ltrasound is a painless procedure increasingly being used in all pregnancies. It has many uses, including determining the stage of pregnancy, detecting twins, and detecting severe fetal malformations (see below).

An ultrasound works by using sound waves to build up a photographic picture of your baby in the uterus. It can be used at any stage during pregnancy. If you are unsure about having ultrasound, talk to your doctor about it.

The scan will show you the outline of your baby's head and body on a screen.

See Week 17
for Amniocentesis

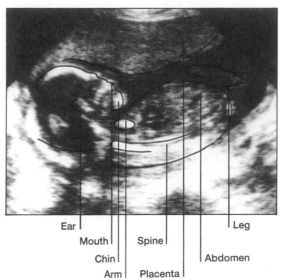

Ear | Leg
Mouth | Spine
Chin | Abdomen
Arm | Placenta

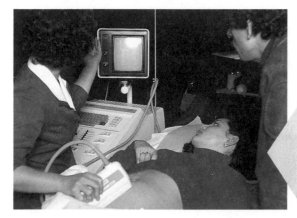

For your ultrasound examination, you lie on a bed and your bare abdomen is smeared with a gel before the scanner is passed over it. Ultrasound is painless (the only requirement being that you have a full bladder) and the results appear immediately on a television screen. Ask for the picture to be explained if you can't tell what's what.

WHAT ULTRASOUND CAN DO

- It determines how old your baby is, which is useful if you are unsure about the date of your last period. If done early in pregnancy this is accurate to within one week.
- It picks up any visible structural abnormalities such as heart, head, spine or kidney conditions.
- It locates the position of the placenta and its condition.
- It detects anything that might make delivery difficult, such as fibroids.

- From around Week 9 an ultrasound scan will be able to detect whether or not you are expecting twins, so be prepared! You will receive special care.

Twins
If you discover that you are expecting twins, you will have to take even greater care of yourself as you will probably get more tired and possibly feel more nauseous. You should take particular care over your

diet. You will also have to plan well ahead to organize two sets of clothes and some equipment such as a double stroller.

The average duration of a twin pregnancy is 36-38 weeks, so you will need to prepare yourself early for labor, which will probably be in the hospital, so have your hospital suitcase packed well before then. It would be worth contacting the National Organization of Mothers of Twins Clubs (see Useful Addresses).

week 17

MON

TUES

WED

THURS

FRI

SAT

SUN

*n*OTES

YOU AND YOUR DEVELOPING BABY

You You may find you are having some pregnancy problems (see Weeks 12 and 13), such as a stuffy nose or an increase in vaginal discharge or that you are sweating more than usual. All these common symptoms of pregnancy will vanish soon after delivery.

Your uterus is expanding quickly; you should now be able to feel the top of it roughly halfway between your pubic bone and your navel (see Week 20). To reduce the possibility of back pain and discomfort later on, take steps to improve your posture (see Week 31).

Baby He can now hear sounds outside your body, which may make him jump. All his limbs are fully formed, as well as his skin and muscles. The chest muscles are starting to make movements similar to those that will be used in respiration. All his joints are able to move and about now you should begin to feel his movements. Tiny fingernails and toenails are beginning to appear.

Your baby measures approximately 7⅛ in (18cm) and now weighs more than the placenta.

Don't forget Note the date when you first feel your baby moving.

*t*ESTS DURING PREGNANCY

*b*y Week 17 you may have had an ultrasound exam (see Week 16) and you will certainly have had routine blood tests. There is another blood test given between Weeks 15 and 20 called the Maternal Serum Alpha-fetoprotein (MSAFP) which is harmless and will give you an indication of possible neural tube defects, such as spina bifida; certain kidney and gastrointestinal problems, threatened miscarriage, and the presence of more than one fetus. If the results are positive, you may be asked to repeat the test or have amniocentesis (see below) which will give you a definite result on one or more possible abnormalities.

See Week 6 for Visiting the doctor.

See Weeks 9 and 10 for Prenatal care.

AMNIOCENTESIS

Amniocentesis is a test carried out to detect certain abnormalities in the fetus. It has to be done at sixteen to eighteen weeks of pregnancy. A sample of the amniotic fluid which surrounds your baby is drawn out and tested for chromosonal abnormalities, such as Down's syndrome, and congenital abnormalities, such as spina bifida.

An ultrasound scan (see Week 16) is always done before the amniocentesis to check the position of the baby and the placenta so that neither is damaged by the needle. However, there is a small chance of an amniocentesis resulting in a miscarriage, so this test is not done on every expectant mother. Talk to your doctor if you are worried.

You have to wait about four weeks for the result of the test which can be a stressful time for you and your partner. If any abnormality is discovered, you will be given the choice of continuing with your pregnancy or terminating it. You may feel there is no point in having amniocentesis if abortion is against your principles, no matter what is wrong with your child.

Amniocentesis is offered to:
● Older women (usually over 35) for whom there is a higher risk of having a baby with Down's syndrome.
● Women who have a family history of Down's syndrome, spina bifida, hemophilia or muscular dystrophy.
● Women whose blood sample has shown a raised alpha-fetoprotein level, suggesting possible fetal abnormalities.
● Women who have already had a handicapped child.

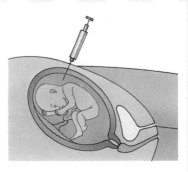

A needle is put through the wall of your abdomen to draw out a sample of amniotic fluid. The fluid is then tested for certain abnormalities.

week 18

month   *date*

MON

TUES

WED

THURS

FRI

SAT

SUN

*n*OTES

YOU AND YOUR DEVELOPING BABY

You If this is your first pregnancy, it is about now that you will probably feel your baby move for the first time. It's an exciting experience you will probably never forget.

If you have flat or 'inverted' (turned in) nipples, it could be a problem in breast-feeding simply because there is little, if anything, for your baby to latch on to. If you are concerned, mention it to your doctor or midwife. Most nipple problems, however, will be quickly remedied by a hungry baby.

Baby Your baby is now beginning to test his reflexes. He is kicking and punching with his well-formed arms and legs and possibly sucking his thumb as well. He is also twisting, turning and wiggling about. Inside his developing lungs tiny air sacs, called alveoli, are starting to form.

Your baby measures about 8in (20cm) in length this week.

Don't forget When buying clothes, think about what the weather will be like in twenty weeks' time.

PREGNANCY WARDROBE

*a*bout now is a good time to go shopping for maternity wear. Earlier than this you may find it depressing seeing those skirts with added flaps and expandable waists: you don't want to imagine the size you will become. Once you've bought some maternity clothes, keep them in the closet for as long as you can and wear them only once they have become necessary, otherwise you'll get bored with them too soon. It makes sense to buy some clothes that you can also wear while breast-feeding, i.e. with front-flaps. But even if you feel like wearing the same clothes day after day, make sure you have one or two outfits you feel good in: it's very important for your morale.

Remember that in summer you will feel very hot and even in winter you won't feel the cold as much as usual: keep to lightweight natural fibers where possible (just increase the number of layers in winter) and wash your clothing often. Clothes should be loose-fitting – around your armholes as well as your waist.

See Week 8 for Looking Good.

Draw attention to your face and away from your middle with necklaces, scarves, collars, brooches and pins. Or draw the eye upwards with bright lipstick, beautiful earrings or a hat.

Dresses Jumpers and smock-style dresses can be worn right throughout your pregnancy. Don't buy dresses with a tight bodice – you won't want your breasts to be restricted. Dresses with a dropped waist can look good but avoid styles with a seam at the waist: they can be unflattering by Week 30.

Shoes Choose shoes that support your feet. Wear low heels throughout your pregnancy. You will find it easiest to stand correctly if your heels are about 1in (2-3cm) high. Avoid high heels: they can throw your weight forward and lead to backache. A long shoe horn will help you to put shoes on in late pregnancy.

Coats Invest in a tent-shaped lightweight raincoat (or a cape, poncho or heavy shawl), and wear it with layers of clothing.

Underwear Wear cotton, not nylon, underwear and make sure it is not too tight. Bikini briefs fit best under your middle. Use a lightweight maternity corset if you feel you need support for your stomach. Wear a support bra from about Week 10 of your pregnancy.

Do not wear garters, elastic-top stockings or tight knee socks: they constrict the legs and can cause varicose veins. Wear support stockings if you have varicose veins.

Slacks Buy slacks with an expandable waist. Leggings are comfortable – wear a large shirt, sweatshirt or T-shirt over them to cover your bottom. Overalls and jumpsuits can be practical though not always flattering.

week 19

month   *date*

MON

___

TUES

___

WED

___

THURS

___

FRI

___

SAT

___

SUN

___

YOU AND YOUR DEVELOPING BABY

You You are probably feeling a lot better and happier these days, especially once your baby's kicking has given you tangible proof of his presence. Share your baby's movements with your partner as soon as you can, though he may not be able to feel them as yet.

Baby This week buds for permanent teeth begin forming behind those that have already developed for the milk teeth. By now your child is drinking a considerable quantity of amniotic fluid each day. At the same time, his stomach is starting to secrete gastric juices, which help him absorb the fluid. After absorption the fluid is filtered by his kidneys and excreted back into the amniotic sac.

Your baby now measures approximately 9in (22.5cm).

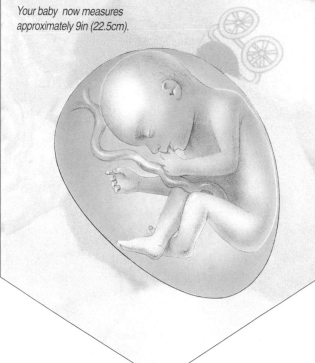

*n*OTES

VITAMINS AND MINERALS

*i*deally, your vitamin and mineral intake will come from food (see Week.3). You should follow a sensible, well-balanced diet. There will be some women who are special cases and they may need additional supplements (see below). Unless prescribed by your doctor, there is no need to take supplements to increase the amounts of vitamins and minerals in your diet. The exception is folic acid, found in raw leafy vegetables and walnuts. This is essential for the development of your baby's central nervous system and you need twice as much during pregnancy. Supplements are supplied free to all pregnant women.

See Week 3 for Healthy Eating

See Week 2 for Safety with Pets

WHAT YOU SHOULD GET FROM YOUR DIET

Vitamins

Vitamin A for resistance to infection, relief of allergies or acne, good vision, formation of tooth enamel, hair and fingernails.
- Dairy products, oily fish, carrots, apricots, tomatoes and greens.

B Vitamins for eye and skin problems, constipation, milk production, infection, bleeding gums, development of healthy red blood cells.
- Whole grains, wheatgerm, beans, nuts, pork, cooked egg yolk, brewer's yeast, milk, hard cheese, mushrooms, potatoes, bananas, green vegetables, oily fish, wholewheat bread.

Vitamin C for absorption of iron, strong and healthy tissues, resistance to infection, building a strong placenta and healing fractures and wounds. May be recommended during pregnancy to help absorb iron.
- Citrus fruits, berry fruits, green, red and yellow raw vegetables, potatoes.

Vitamin D for absorption of calcium and phosphorous, and building strong bones.
- Found in oily fish, dairy products and sunlight on skin.

Vitamin E for improved circulation and hormone production.
- Most foods, especially wheatgerm, eggs.

Vitamin K Helps your blood to clot.
- Green vegetables and alfalfa sprouts.

Minerals

Calcium Needed for the development of strong bones and teeth in your baby. It also enables your blood to clot and your muscles to work smoothly. You need almost twice as much calcium during pregnancy and breast-feeding, especially in the first four months of pregnancy. Vitamin D is essential for the efficient absorption of calcium.
- Leafy vegetables, cauliflower, fish, oranges, dairy foods, whole grains, beans and nuts.

Iron Needed in the formation of hemoglobin for your increased number of red blood cells. Vitamin C helps your body absorb iron. You need about twice as much iron during pregnancy and your doctor may prescribe it for you.
- Cooked egg yolk, sardines, whole grains, dark green leaf vegetables, raisins, prunes, nuts, dark molasses.

Salt Needed in pregnancy because the salt in your blood is diluted by increased body fluids.

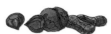

SPECIAL CASES FOR SUPPLEMENTS

- Women pregnant during adolescence (they are still growing themselves).
- Women who are underweight or run down or who were eating an unbalanced diet when they became pregnant.
- Women who were overweight when they became pregnant.

- Women on a strict diet, such as macrobiotics.
- Women who are allergic to certain vital foods, such as cow's milk or wheat.
- Women who have previously lost a baby from miscarriage or stillbirth.
- Women who have had three pregnancies in two years.

- Women suffering from chronic diseases for which they take continuous medication.
- Women who have a multiple pregnancy.
- Women who have to work particularly hard or who are under a lot of stress.
- Women who smoke, drink or take drugs.

week 20

MON

TUES

WED

THURS

FRI

SAT

SUN

*n*OTES

YOU AND YOUR DEVELOPING BABY

You Your uterus presses up against your lungs and pushes your stomach outwards so you begin to look more pregnant. Your naval may be starting to flatten or pop out – it will stay that way until after delivery.

Baby Your baby is growing rapidly and now measures approximately 10in (25.5cm), roughly half of what the average baby measures at birth. His weight is around 12oz (340g). His growth will soon slow down a little. His muscles are increasing in strength and active movements can now be felt. They may feel like light flutters or like bubbles bursting against your abdomen.

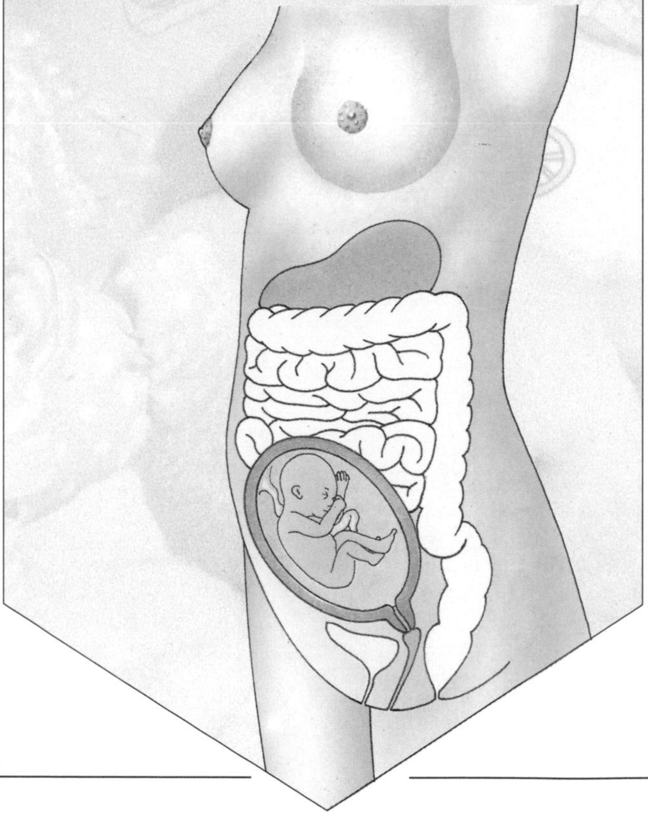

*t*he fundus is the top of your uterus and its height is a gauge used by your doctor during an examination to see how far advanced your pregnancy is. It is normally measured in centimeters from your pubic bone to below your breastbone.

In order to accommodate your growing baby your uterus will have to increase its volume about 1,000-fold during pregnancy and, as it does, it will take up the space of other organs. This can lead to some of the problems of later pregnancy, such as breathlessness, constipation, heartburn and frequency of urination.

On average a non-pregnant uterus is roughly the size of a tangerine. By six weeks it is the size of a small apple and two weeks later that of a large orange. At Week 14 it looks like a small melon. At full term it can measure as much as 15in (38cm) in length, 10in (25.5cm) in width and 8in (20cm) from front to back. The weight of the uterus itself increases during pregnancy by approximately twenty times, from a pre-pregnant weight of 1½oz (40g) to almost 2lb (800g), at its heaviest, immediately after the baby is born.

With your first child, a phenomenon called 'lightening' may occur after Week 36 which means that your baby drops slightly and engages in your pelvis. This will put pressure on your groin and pelvis. With a second or subsequent baby, this may not happen until the onset of labor.

You will probably notice your uterus expanding after Week 12 when it becomes too large to stay hidden in your pelvis. From then on it enlarges at a regular rate until Week 36 when it reaches to just below your breastbone. This may make it awkward to breathe and you may feel a jabbing pain in your ribcage.

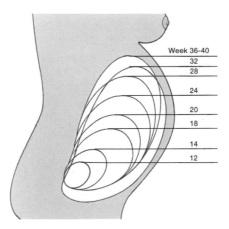

Week 36-40
32
28
24
20
18
14
12

PRE-ECLAMPSIA

Pre-eclampsia is a possible condition of later pregnancy involving raised blood pressure and protein in your urine; it rarely occurs before Week 20. It usually develops slowly and there is a risk to both you and your unborn baby if it goes unnoticed. This is one of the reasons why it is important to go to all your prenatal visits so that your blood pressure and urine can be tested.

It is best to prevent pre-eclampsia, but if it develops and is severe you may have to go to the hospital for bedrest, sedation and monitoring of the kidney function and blood pressure. It will disappear completely once your baby is born. Your doctor will be looking out for:
● swelling of the feet, ankles, face and hands due to fluid retention;
● raised blood pressure;
● protein in your urine (this is why you give a urine sample at every prenatal visit);
● excessive weight gain.

week 21

month   *date*

MON

_____

TUES

_____

WED

_____

THURS

_____

FRI

_____

SAT

_____

SUN

_____

*n*OTES

YOU AND YOUR DEVELOPING BABY

You Around now you will probably be starting to feel energetic, healthy and very positive – in short, better than you have ever felt before. Remember to rest even if you don't feel like it. You may be feeling constantly hungry as well. The next ten weeks is when you put on about half of the weight you gain during pregnancy (see Week 25) so watch what you eat. Eat well – but not for two.

Baby Around now your baby's skin becomes opaque. White blood cells are starting to be manufactured, which play an important part in fighting disease and infection. Your child's tongue is now fully developed, and, if female, her internal organs of reproduction – the vagina and the womb – have formed. Your baby's legs are now in proportion with the rest of his body.

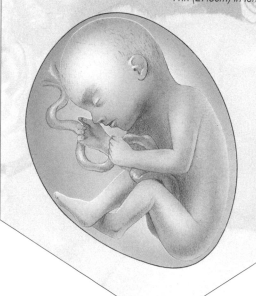

Your baby weighs around 1lb (450g) and measures about 11in (27.5cm) in length.

$\mathcal{Y}$ou may find that your nesting instinct is very strong during pregnancy and you are happiest staying in your home environment. But if it is your first child you're probably only too aware that this may be your last opportunity for a vacation alone together for a while. Try to plan an enjoyable but essentially restful vacation: relax by a pool or escape to the countryside. Enjoy the company of your partner.

When is the best time to go away?

First trimester   Nausea, vomiting and tiredness may stop you from enjoying any travel. If you have to travel, do so in that part of the day when you feel best.

Second trimester   This is the best time to go away during pregnancy – especially between Weeks 20 and 27 – although you may still get uncomfortable and restless if you have to sit in cramped conditions on a trip. Walk around as much as you can to keep your circulation going. Your feet may swell on plane trips.

Third trimester   It is advisable not to go on any long trips toward the end of pregnancy. You probably won't feel like it. In your 9th month, airlines will not deny you boarding domestic or international flights. But they do advise you consult with your doctor prior to the flight.

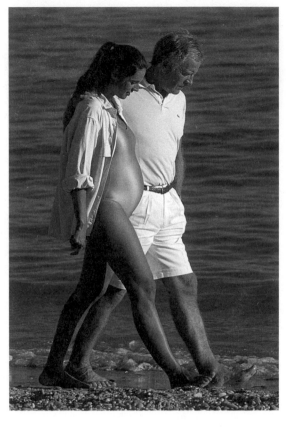

See Week 15
for Pelvic Floor
Exercises

See Week 22
for Keeping Fit

VACATION PRECAUTIONS

Do's

● Talk to your doctor if you want to go away for longer than a month at any stage of your pregnancy.
● Take your medical records with you if necessary.
● Get the name and number of a doctor in the place where you're going, just in case of emergency.
● Check with the doctor that you are allowed to have any vaccinations you may need.
● Work out a timetable allowing for delays. You won't feel like rushing.
● Travel by train rather than by car for long distances – it's more comfortable.

Don'ts

● Don't travel unless absolutely necessary in the first three months if you have had bleeding early in pregnancy or a previous miscarriage.
● Don't take drugs to prevent sea or air sickness without consulting your doctor.
● Don't undertake long car journeys (three hours or more) unless accompanied by another driver.
● Don't eat too much unfamiliar food abroad, and drink bottled, not local water.
● Don't go on a strenuous sports vacations.

week 22

MON

TUES

WED

THURS

FRI

SAT

SUN

YOU AND YOUR DEVELOPING BABY

You You will probably notice that your baby is developing a pattern of waking and sleeping and may well be at his most active while you are wanting to sleep. At this stage his kicks are endearing, and still quite gentle.

You may find that you are bringing up small amounts of acid fluid; antacid tablets will help neutralize this. Your gums may bleed more than usual (see Week 8).

Baby By the end of the fifth month vernix, a greasy, white, cheesy-looking substance, is beginning to form on your child's skin. Vernix is a mixture of sebum, from the sebaceous glands, and skin cells. It protects your baby's delicate, newly formed skin from the possible damage of living in liquid for nine months. The vernix adheres to the lanugo all over the skin and although most of it will have disappeared before birth, some is left to lubricate your baby's passage along the birth canal during delivery.

Your baby has now grown to about 11½in (29cm) long and weighs about 1lb 2oz (500g).

*n*OTES

Don't forget Go and see your dentist if you haven't already.

*e*ven if you dislike exercising, try and keep active during pregnancy as you will feel more comfortable. A brisk walk or an occasional swim is enough – the only essential exercise is your pelvic floor exercises (see Week 15).

If you enjoy exercising, find out what is available in your area. There may be classes run by your local hospital or even swimming classes for pregnant women at your local Y. Here are some gentle exercises to do at home.

If you have had a previous miscarriage or are experiencing any complications check with your doctor before exercising during the first three months of pregnancy.

Do all exercises slowly up to ten times each, unless suggested otherwise. Carry them out rhythmically – never jerkily – and relax for a minute or two after completing each one.

Never strain yourself and don't exercise until you drop or are in pain – you're not training for the Olympics. Never do sit-ups or raise both legs simultaneously while lying down when you are pregnant. Either can damage your abdominal muscles and strain your back.

Keep breathing at a controlled pace and try to relax the parts of your body that are not being exercised. Arrange pillows where necessary to keep comfortable and always get up from the floor by rolling onto your side and using your arms to push you up. After you have carried out your exercises, lie on your back and rest for a few minutes.

See Week 15 for Pelvic Floor Exercises

See Week 30 for Learning Relaxation

See Week 31 for Good Posture

HIP STRETCHING

Sit upright on the floor with your back straight (or lean against a wall).

1 With the soles of your feet together, and your heels as near to your body as possible, gently push your knees towards the floor. If this is difficult, push one knee first and then the other.

2 Keeping your legs flat on the floor, move them as far apart as you can. You should feel your groin stretching.

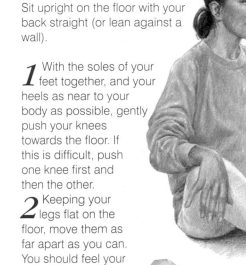

STOMACH MUSCLES

1 Lie on your back with your knees bent and your feet flat on the floor. Have a pillow under your head and shoulders. Tighten your stomach muscles so that your abdomen is gently pulled down towards your back. Hold for three seconds, then relax slowly. (This exercise is also good for regaining your figure after birth.)

2 Keeping the small of your back pressed down, slowly stretch both legs until they are straight. Draw one knee back up, and then the other, without lifting the small of your back off the floor. If your back hurts at any point, stop. Otherwise repeat until you can do the exercise ten times.

(Continued in Week 23)

week 23

month   *date*

MON

TUES

WED

THURS

FRI

SAT

SUN

YOU AND YOUR DEVELOPING BABY

You You may have already noticed a painless, though uncomfortable, hardening of your stomach which occurs roughly every twenty minutes and lasts for about twenty seconds. This is a 'Braxton Hicks' uterine contraction; they occur all the way through pregnancy, although they are not usually noticeable before this stage. They help your uterus grow and ensure a good circulation of blood through your uterine vessels.

You may also sometimes get a stitch-like pain down the side of your belly, which is your uterine muscle stretching. Have a rest and the pain will go.

Baby Your baby is now moving vigorously, often in response to touch and sound. A loud noise nearby may make him jump and kick. He is also swallowing small amounts of amniotic fluid and passing tiny amounts of urine back into it. Sometimes he may get hiccups and you can feel the jerk of each hiccup.

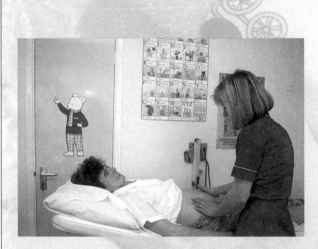

The doctor or midwife feels your abdomen to work out the baby's position so she can listen to his heartbeat.

*n*OTES

*b*elow are some more exercises for you to do to strengthen breasts, back and the pelvic area; remember to exercise gently and read the advice in Week 22 before you start.

Squatting makes your pelvic joints more flexible and stretches and strengthens thighs and back muscles. It can also relieve back pain.

Swimming is wonderful exercise for pregnancy. Even if you can't swim you can exercise by holding on to the side of the pool, with your back to the wall, and cycling in the water.

See Week 31 for Good Posture

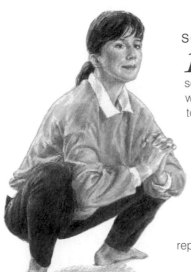

SQUATTING

1 **Full squats**   Keeping your back straight, and legs apart, squat down low. Distribute your weight evenly between heels and toes. To stretch further, press elbows against inner thighs.

2 **Half squats**   Hold onto a chair and place your right foot in front of your left. Point your right knee slightly out and slowly bend both knees. Keep your bottom tucked in and back straight. Stand up slowly, then repeat with the other leg in front.

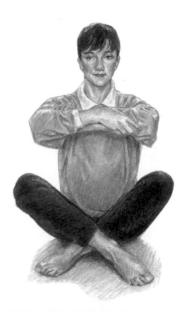

BREAST MUSCLES

1 Sit cross-legged on the floor with your back straight. Bend your arms and grip your left wrist with your right hand and vice versa. Breathe in and blow out once. Now breathe in, hold your breath and push your shoulders and ribcage down.

2 Tip your chin gently onto your chest and slide each wrist gently towards your elbows ten times. Then raise your head and blow out slowly. Repeat once. If you find you can't hold your breath for so long, build up to it slowly.

BACK STRENGTHENING

1 **Pelvic rock**   Lie on your back with your feet together, flat on the floor, and knees slightly bent. Place a hand under the hollow of your back. Using your stomach muscles, press your spine against the floor until your back is flat. Relax and repeat.

2 **The cat**   Get on all fours with your hands and knees apart. Arch your back gently and push your head down so you feel a stretch from neck to tail. Now raise your head as you relax your back to its normal position. Repeat once.

week 24

month   *date*

MON

TUES

WED

THURS

FRI

SAT

SUN

YOU AND YOUR DEVELOPING BABY

You You may begin to put on weight fairly rapidly and your feet will probably start to feel the strain. Check that your shoes are comfortable and give you enough support; go barefoot at home if you feel like it. Rest with your feet up – preferably above your heart – whenever possible.

If you are finding your job more exhausting try to work part-time, from early in the third trimester (from Week 28 on) if your employer agrees.

Baby Your baby is still rather thin and his skin quite wrinkled because he has not yet laid down deposits of fat, but he is growing lengthwise. His arms and legs now have a normal amount of muscle and they are moving vigorously. Creases are appearing on his palms and fingertips. His eyelids have separated and he can open his eyes.

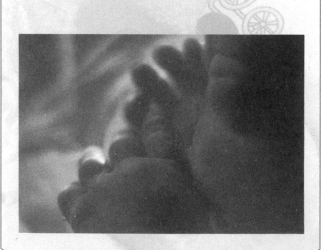

Your baby's hands are active at this time. This muscular coordination is sufficiently developed for him to suck his thumb!

*n*OTES

*t*HE FATHER'S ROLE

*Y*our partner is no doubt as pleased as you are about your pregnancy and the future baby. He will also be concerned, although his anxieties may well be different from yours. He may worry about how your relationship will change, about how his life will be disrupted and, if you are giving up work, about whether he is going to be able to support you both financially. It may also be difficult at first for him to realize that a baby is really there; it can feel strange being so closely involved with the pregnancy and yet in a sense so removed.

Include him as much as possible. Let him feel the baby kicking, invite him along to doctor's appointments, prenatal classes and, of course, the birth – but don't be upset if he feels he doesn't want to come.

Explain to your partner how you are feeling, because your emotions will be changing more than usual. It may be difficult for him to keep pace. Make sure you apologize if you find yourself snapping at him. Try and get him to help out in your daily routine if you are feeling sick or too tired to do anything.

Your partner may feel jealous both of the coming child and of your ability to nurture new life within you. He may also dislike being the supporting actor rather than the star and may feel he is only peripherally helpful. Partners need both physical and mental reassurance. Even if you don't feel like sex, cuddle and caress him, and try not to let the pillows that surround your body in bed every night get in between you too much! Try and talk to your partner about his emotions and worries, even if you feel more like concentrating on yourself.

See Week 38 for Fathers in Labor

See Weeks 15 for Sex during Pregnancy

See Week 14 for Other Children

Be positive and appreciative: let your partner know she is doing her best. Try to be sympathetic and supportive – show her you love her and help her where you can. If at times you feel left out, rest assured that what you are sharing will bond the two of you closer together all your lives. Read all you can about pregnancy and childbirth, and prepare yourself for adjustments afterwards.

PRACTICAL CHECKLIST FOR FATHERS

- Do you know the quickest route to the hospital, the correct entrance and where you can park?
- Have you visited the hospital beforehand to see where the delivery rooms, canteen and wards are?
- Do you know what the signs of labor are? (See Week 37)
- Have you discussed how your partner feels about pain relief? (See Week 35)
- If you plan to attend the birth, are you as knowledgeable about it as your partner?
- Are the relevant numbers displayed by the phone?

week 25

month _____ *date* _____

MON
_____

TUES
_____

WED
_____

THURS
_____

FRI
_____

SAT
_____

SUN
_____

*n*OTES

YOU AND YOUR DEVELOPING BABY

You Around now is the best time in pregnancy for many women. Make the most of it. You may find that you are looking flushed with the increase in blood circulation underneath your skin. You should also be feeling happy and contented; if you are not, try and talk about it to your partner, friends and your doctor.

The minus side is that you may be experiencing some of the problems of pregnancy, such as backache, cramps and need to urinate more often. Your heart and lungs are now doing fifty per cent more work than usual and you will find that you are sweating more because of your raised body fluid levels.

Baby Your baby's bone centers are beginning to harden. He will be fattening out, so that his eyes seem less hollow in his head.

Growing at a steady pace, your baby now measures about 1ft 2in (35cm) and weighs around 1lb 14oz (850g).

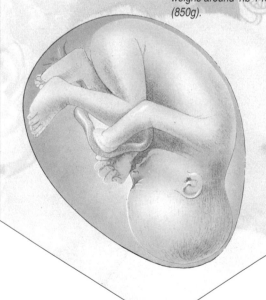

*a*t one stage it was thought that pregnant women should 'eat for two'. Then opinions changed and women were advised that they should try not to gain weight during pregnancy as it would stay with them forever. Today, studies show that underweight women are probably at greater risk of bearing low-birth-weight babies and that a steady weight gain is desirable. You will be weighed each time you go to the doctor's, partly to show that your baby is growing normally and partly to check on your own health: a sudden change up or down in weight could signify problems. If you are putting on too much weight it could indicate pre-eclampsia (see Week 20). Dieting and cutting down on fluids will not help, so continue to eat well.

The diagram above shows how your weight gain is made up. However much weight you put on during pregnancy, you will gain roughly a quarter of the total between Weeks 12 and 20, half between Weeks 20 and 30 and the last quarter between Weeks 30 and 38. If you find your weight shooting up at the end, this is probably due to water retention, so don't worry. You will lose it all after your baby is born, although it follows that the less weight you put on, the easier this will be lost.

If you are worried about your weight, discuss it with your doctor; do not start dieting during pregnancy. You can do more harm to yourself and your baby by eating too little of the foods you need than by eating too much.

Baby 39%
Placenta 9%
Breasts 8%
Amniotic fluid 11%
Uterus 11%
Blood 22%

See Week 3 for Healthy Eating

See Week 19 for Vitamins and Minerals

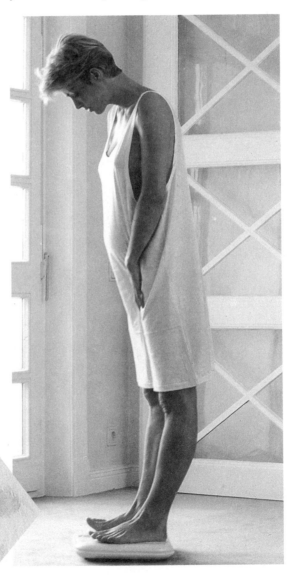

Most women gain about 30lb (13.5kg) altogether during pregnancy and find that they are 7-14lb (3-6kg) heavier after giving birth than before they became pregnant. The amount varies between individuals and in one woman from one pregnancy to the next.

week 26

MON

TUES

WED

THURS

FRI

SAT

SUN

*n*OTES

YOU AND YOUR DEVELOPING BABY

You Take advantage of your surplus energy and any spare time to start preparing for your child's arrival. Get organized: make lists of anything you need to do around your home and any clothes and other equipment you need to buy.

Baby The branches of your baby's lungs (the bronchi) are now developing, but his lungs will not be fully formed until after he is born. His head is now in better proportion to his body. Fat stores are beginning to accumulate.

Your baby now weighs about 2lb (900g) and measures around 1ft 2in (36cm).

*S*ome minor problems, or discomforts; start in early pregnancy and continue until the last few months (see Weeks 12 and 13). Others only begin towards, or during, the final trimester. You may, of course, experience few, or none, of them.

Most of these problems are to do with your uterus squeezing out your other organs. If any of these problems prevent you from getting enough rest at night, nap during the day. If any of them worry you, then talk to your doctor or midwife and call your doctor if you have any swelling in the hands and feet, a high fever, persistent headache or severe cramps.

See Weeks 12 and 13 for Common Problems

Backache See Week 31.

Breathlessness From about Week 30 you might find breathing difficult, due to pressure on your diaphragm from your growing uterus. It will become easier once your baby's head has engaged. Remember to sit up or stand as straight as possible, and prop a few pillows under your head and shoulders in bed. If you have chest pain or swelling, consult your doctor.

Discomfort in bed This could be due to indigestion or heartburn, or to pressure from your enlarged uterus. If your mattress is not firm, place a board under it. Distribute pillows under different parts of your body until you get comfortable.

Incontinence You may leak a little urine when you cough, laugh or bend down. This could be due to your enlarged uterus pressing on your bladder, or to weak pelvic floor muscles (see Week 15). Empty your bladder often and avoid lifting anything heavy; exercise your pelvic floor.

Indigestion and heartburn Some of the foods you normally enjoy may give you indigestion. If you can work out what they are, avoid them. Eat smaller meals and sit up straight when eating to take the pressure off your stomach.

Heartburn is a burning pain in the lower part of your chest, throat, back of your mouth or stomach, often accompanied by the regurgitation of sour fluid. It is caused by the relaxation of a stomach valve, allowing acid to pass into the tube.

Sleep with your shoulders well propped up. A glass of milk before sleeping may help. Don't sit slumped in a chair and try not to bend down, putting your head below your chest; avoid rich, fried or spicy foods; and wear clothes that are loose at the waist.

Nausea Nausea towards the end of pregnancy may be due to the pressure of your uterus on your stomach. Eat small frequent meals.

Pelvic discomfort You may develop pain around your pubic area, or in your groin and down the inside of your thighs. This could be caused by your baby's head pressing on nerves, or by your pelvic joints softening in preparation for labor. Don't stand or sit for long periods and avoid violent exercise. Rest frequently and take the occasional acetaminophen tablet if the pain gets too uncomfortable.

'Pins and needles' This is due to the increase in body fluid exerting pressure on your nerves and tendons. Hold your hands above your head and wiggle your fingers.

Rib pain After about Week 30, when the top of the uterus is high, you may feel a pain just below your breasts. You will feel most comfortable sitting on a straight chair or lying down flat. Stretch upwards to lift your ribcage off your uterus.

Swelling of legs, ankles, fingers (Edema) Edema is an increase in fluid retention in your body, especially in the lower limbs. This is due to the pressure of the uterus on the vessels that return blood from the lower parts of your body to the heart. You may notice your shoes feeling tight, your ankles becoming wrinkled and your rings not fitting – remove them. Mention this to your doctor in case it is a sign of pre-eclampsia (see Week 20). Avoid standing for too long, sit down wherever you can, and rest with your feet raised above your heart. It may help to wear maternity support stockings. Avoid garters or tight socks or shoes.

week 27

MON

TUES

WED

THURS

FRI

SAT

SUN

YOU AND YOUR DEVELOPING BABY

You You are probably beginning to put on weight at a steady rate and may be aware that you are starting to get more tired. You may notice quite regular Braxton Hicks contractions now, especially when walking. Try wearing a lightweight maternity corset if you feel it would help. Keep exercising. You should now be able to feel the top of your uterus about halfway between your navel and your breast bone.

Baby Your baby's eyes are almost always blue or dark blue at this stage as the eye coloring is not fully developed until a few months after birth. Occasionally, however, a baby's eyes turn brown within only a few hours of him being born.

Don't forget Buy an approved infant car seat for the ride home from the hospital.

*n*OTES

58

PREPARING FOR BABY

*i*t is not essential that your baby has a room of his own: he can equally well share with older siblings or with you. If he's to share your bedroom it is a good idea to keep him in a separate corner so you will have some privacy.

Even if he can have his own room there is no need to spend a lot of money on equipment or totally redecorating the room. Your child will be happiest sleeping and playing in a room in which he can relax and enjoy himself – and that won't happen if you worry about him ruining the decor. Remember that he will grow quickly and his requirements will constantly be changing.

Whether you are preparing the room from scratch or adapting a room, there are several things to consider. Remember to incorporate safety features now in preparation for a crawling – and later, walking – baby.

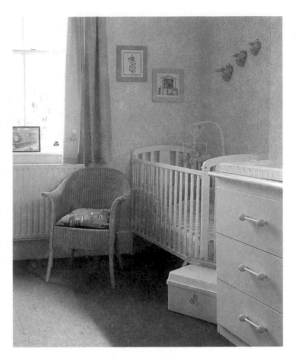

See Weeks 28 and 29 for Shopping for Baby Furniture and Equipment

See Week 33 for Getting Ready

Comfort A rocking chair or a low, comfortable chair is ideal for feeding and comforting a baby – you will also need a few cushions for behind your back and to rest your baby on.

Peace A dimmer switch or night-light or a thick lampshade on a lamp is ideal for night feeding and checking your baby without waking him. Cover all unused sockets with special childproof covers.

Temperature Indoor temperatures should be kept at between 68° to 72°F. Remember babies' ability to regulate their own body temperature is immature; in addition, they don't have much in the way of body fat to insulate them. If you are using an approved, UL labeled space heater or heating stove in your child's room, be sure to turn it off before going to bed. Consider installing a humidifier or buying a portable one if the air gets too dry.

Windows Make sure your windows and doors are draft-proof or that your baby does not sleep too close to them. Guard low windows with close-spaced vertical bars (removable in case of fire).

Furniture Furniture should be sufficiently heavy so it cannot be pulled over. Wooden furniture should be painted with non-toxic (i.e. no-lead) paint. You will need drawer space for clothes and storage space for diapers. A chest of drawers with the top at waist height might double as a changing table.

Dust If asthma is a family problem, you probably know what to do. Avoid woollen carpets, rugs and blankets and make sure all surfaces are as easy to clean as possible.

Crib position Your baby should sleep in a well-ventilated room far removed from areas where people might smoke. You should not give him a pillow or a crib bumper at this stage, nor should he sleep on a sheepskin. These sensible precautions will help to reduce the risk of crib death (Sudden Infant Death Syndrome or SIDS). Another precaution is to place the baby on his back or side whether in his crib or carriage until he is old enough to choose his own sleeping position.

week 28

MON

TUES

WED

THURS

FRI

SAT

SUN

*n*OTES

YOU AND YOUR DEVELOPING BABY

You Week 28 is the first week of your third and last trimester, which often seems the longest. Some of the minor problems of pregnancy, such as indigestion and cramps, may have become a part of life but be assured they will disappear after the birth. Get as much rest and sleep as possible and keep up your calcium intake by eating more milk, cheese or yogurt. ·

Baby Your baby's lungs are reaching maturity and although he might have breathing problems and difficulty keeping himself warm if born, with modern special care facilities he has a chance of survival.

By now your baby is large enough for his position in your uterus to be assessed during an abdominal examination. He may still be in the breech or transverse (sideways) position (see Understanding your Notes, page 88) though most babies turn head down by Week 36.

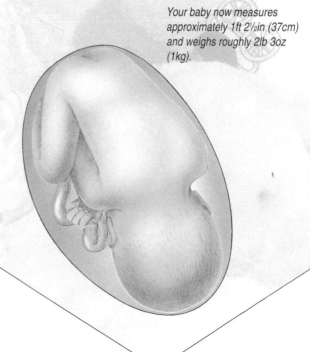

Your baby now measures approximately 1ft 2½in (37cm) and weighs roughly 2lb 3oz (1kg).

SLEEPING EQUIPMENT

it is a good idea to shop for equipment and baby clothes at this stage, while you still have the energy. You will feel tired and uncomfortable in the later stages of pregnancy and there will be little time when the baby is born. If you feel it is 'tempting fate' to fill the house with baby things before he is even born, most stores will let you order major pieces of equipment now, provided you leave a deposit, and will deliver them to your home after the birth. Or buy from shops that will let you return unused goods – and keep all your receipts.

If this is your first baby it can be difficult to know exactly what you will need and the choice can be baffling. If this is your second child, you'll have a better idea of your needs. The suggestions below and in Week 29 will help you to make decisions. If you're buying new equipment, make sure that it complies with U.S. Consumer Product safety regulations.

See Week 29 for Equipment for Transporting Baby

See Week 33 for First Baby Clothes

BUYING THE BEDDING

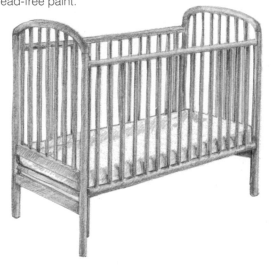

Crib You don't need a full-size crib at first but something smaller, such as a bassinet, Moses basket, or carriage.

If you borrow or inherit a used crib, check with the U.S. Consumer Product Safety Commission Hotline (1-800-638-2772) to make sure it hasn't been recalled. Make sure that the distance between the slats is no greater than $2^3/_8$ inches and the corner posts are less than $^5/_8$ inches tall. There should be at least 26 inches from the top of the rail to the mattress set at its lowest level. Check that there are no splinters or sharp parts anywhere and that it is painted only with lead-free paint.

Some cribs convert into a junior bed later.

Crib mattress The most important thing is that the mattress fit the crib snugly leaving no space around the edges. Never use a plastic garbage bag to cover the mattress.

Bedding You will need at least three fitted crib sheets. Crib bumpers must be secured tightly with no loose strings or straps. He must not use a pillow for at least the first year, but he will need blankets. Several light layers (preferably, open weave blankets) are warmer and safer than one heavy one; avoid fringes which your baby may suck.

Baby monitor This will let you hear the baby crying if you live in a large or noisy house. You can get one that has a battery-operated receiver so you can take it from room to room.

week 29

MON

TUES

WED

THURS

FRI

SAT

SUN

*n*OTES

YOU AND YOUR DEVELOPING BABY

You In the bath you may be able to watch your baby move from one side of your abdomen to another. His hand movements are softer than his rather jerky knee and foot movements.

If you haven't already done so, go for a swim. You will enjoy feeling much lighter than you do normally. You may start needing to sit down often and you probably won't feel like running around.

Baby Your baby has filled almost all the space in your uterus and his head is now more or less in proportion with his body. Although he may still be lying with his head up, within a few weeks he should have turned upside down and will then appear to fit more comfortably. He is growing at a weekly rate of just under $3/_8$in (1cm) and now measures around 1ft 3in (38cm).

Your baby is gaining about 7oz (200g) a week and now weighs about 2lb 4oz (1.02kg).

Don't forget Begin to delegate chores to anyone who offers.

&QUIPMENT FOR TRANSPORTING BABY

*Y*our lifestyle and budget are important factors when deciding what equipment to buy to transport your baby. If you drive everywhere, then your needs will be different than if you travel on public transportation or walk to do your shopping. A large carriage is ideal in rural areas but is obviously not suitable if you live up flights of stairs, for example. Nowadays there are many collapsible and adjustable carriages and strollers (many with shopping trays), car safety seats, cloth baby carriers and slings to choose from.

CHOOSING THE RIGHT EQUIPMENT

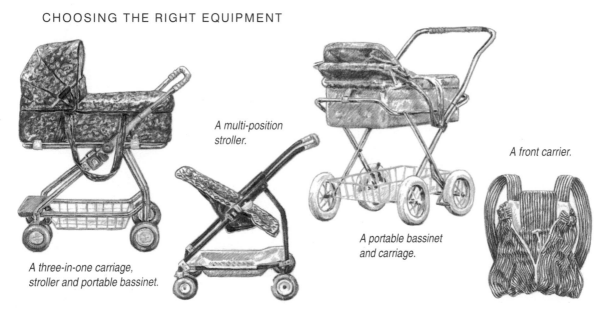

A multi-position stroller.

A front carrier.

A portable bassinet and carriage.

A three-in-one carriage, stroller and portable bassinet.

Carriage When choosing a carriage, check that it is light enough for you to push easily, that the handles are at a comfortable height and that the brakes can be operated without letting go of the handle. Make sure that there is a mattress and check that a shopping basket can be fitted without interfering with the brakes. Make sure there are anchor points for a safety harness. Check that you'll be able to get it through your front door. With a second hand carriage, make sure the tires are not worn, that there are no nuts loose or missing and that the brakes work properly.
Carriage harness Buy one that is strong and washable and easy to fasten and unfasten.
Carriage net This will keep off insects and cats.
Strollers Newborn babies shouldn't travel in upright or even semi-upright strollers as their back muscles are not strong enough to support them sitting up. The most useful stroller has a seat that can be put into several positions, and that can face both forwards and backwards. Check that the stroller is light enough to carry easily and see how simple it is to fold with one hand – imagine holding a baby in the other.
Baby carrier or sling Your baby will enjoy being held close to you and it leaves your hands free.

Check that it has adjustable straps and a head support.
Car safety seat All states now require that babies and young children be restrained while traveling by car. When acquiring a safety seat be certain it has a label indicating that it meets or exceeds Federal Motor Vehicle Safety Standard (FMVSS) 213. For more information, contact the National Highway & Traffic Safety Administration (see Useful Addresses). But first, check your car's owner manual for instructions on proper installation of a child restraint. Convertible car seats which can be used for infants and toddlers can be more economical in the long run.

See Week 28 for Sleeping Equipment

See Week 33 for First Baby Clothes

week 30

YOU AND YOUR DEVELOPING BABY

You From now on you will become much larger, slower and clumsier. You may feel as if all your internal organs are being squeezed out and put under pressure from your enlarging uterus.

Baby Your baby is probably lying in a curled-up position with his knees bent, his arms and legs crossed and his chin resting on his chest. He now begins to move less and to settle. Most babies adopt a head downwards position so that they can be born head first. If your baby is one of the four per cent who has his bottom first ('breech' presentation), or even rarer, is lying sideways (transverse), he may still turn in the next six weeks.

notes

Don't forget If you haven't already done so, stop smoking now. Your baby needs oxygen to enable him to grow and smoking reduces the amount he will get.

*L*EARNING RELAXATION

elaxing is all about releasing the tension in your body and in your mind. Being able to relax will help you during labor to counteract the natural response to pain, which is to tense your muscles and hold your breath. Once you can relax both during and between contractions, you will be able to work with them.

Many organizations sponsor prenatal, or before childbirth, educational classes designed to prepare you and your partner for the birth (see below). As part of many of these classes you learn breathing and relaxation techniques, such as the Lamaze and Bradley methods and newer approaches, to help you deal with labor pains. The weekly classes usually start eight to ten weeks before your baby is due. You should also visit the hospital maternity ward to become familiar with the surroundings.

See Week 34 for Breathing for Labor

PREPARING YOURSELF

Physical relaxation Start by getting comfortable. Either sit or lie but arrange pillows around you so that every bit of your body is supported. Begin with your toes. First tense up all of the muscles in your toes and then relax them, letting them go so that they are all floppy. Then tense your feet – and let go.

Continue on up your body: your calves, thighs, buttocks, stomach and so on, right up to your face, tensing and then relaxing every single part. This should take about five minutes. Then do it again, this time beginning from the top. Continue on until your whole body is as floppy as a rag doll.

Mental relaxation Get comfortable and clear your mind of anything that's making you nervous. Then concentrate on your breathing: breathe in deeply, hold your breath for a count of five seconds, and then breathe out slowly. As you do so, make sure all your muscles are relaxed – drop your shoulders and jaw, and unclench your hands – and continue to breathe deeply.

Then let your imagination flow. Picture yourself on a beach in the sun under a blue sky, hearing the gentle noise of the waves beside you, or imagine you are floating up to the clouds. Choose whatever image appeals to you.

Where to go Childbirth preparation classes are offered by most hospitals, by local affiliates of the International Childbirth Education Association (ICEA) (see Useful Addresses), and by local birthing centers and home-birth organizations.

Some classes are in the evening for fathers and working women. The advantage of going to classes run by the hospital where you are planning on delivering is that you will meet local expectant mothers and nurse/midwives who can familiarize you with that particular institution.

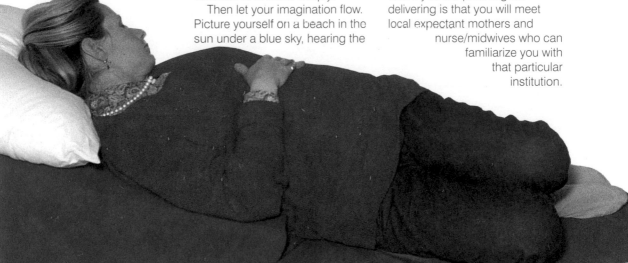

65

week 31

MON

_____

TUES

_____

WED

_____

THURS

_____

FRI

_____

SAT

_____

SUN

_____

NOTES

YOU AND YOUR DEVELOPING BABY

You You are probably beginning to feel breathless when you overdo things, which may make you become impatient for the birth. Or, you may find yourself becoming completely absorbed with your body and your baby's movements. It can be quite a dilemma. Just take care if you do find yourself withdrawing from the world around you. Make sure you don't let your partner feel left out.

If your breasts are becoming heavy, begin wearing a well-fitting bra at night as well as during the day from now on. Good support will make them feel more comfortable.

Baby As your baby grows plumper, his skin fills out and becomes smoother. Both the vernix and the lanugo begin to disappear.

This week your baby measures around 1ft 3½in (39cm) and weighs about 3lb 2oz (1.4kg).

Don't forget Never stand up when you can sit, and never sit when you can lie down.

good POSTURE

See Week 26 for Discomfort in Bed

backache can occur at any time during pregnancy, though the greatest risk is now. If your stomach muscles are not strong enough to carry your extra weight, your back muscles are forced to work to support your spine. This puts strain on them. It helps to stand, sit and lie properly. Backache can also be caused by the way the baby lies in the uterus.

When standing Always stand as straight as possible and don't lean backwards. Improve your posture by wearing low (or flat) heels, tucking your buttocks in, keeping your shoulders dropped and carrying yourself as if you want the top of your head to touch the ceiling. Avoid stooping; instead kneel, sit or squat.

When sitting Sit well back in a chair and support your back by putting a rolled-up towel or small cushion in the hollow of your spine.

When lying down Use a firm mattress and lie flat on your back or on your side. Support your body with pillows wherever they are needed – if lying on your side, try placing them under your head and upper arm; under your stomach; under your top knee and under your hips. To ease upper backache, lie flat on your back with pillows under your head and knees (provided you are comfortable lying flat on your back).

Lifting and carrying Avoid lifting anything heavy if you can. If you need to carry heavy items, keep them close to your body. Distribute the weight evenly: put shopping in two bags of equal weight and carry one in either hand rather than a single heavy one making you lopsided.

Low backache To relieve your spine of your baby's weight, get on all fours as often as possible. Do the cat exercise (see Week 23) whenever you can and, if you feel like it, you could scrub the kitchen floor daily.

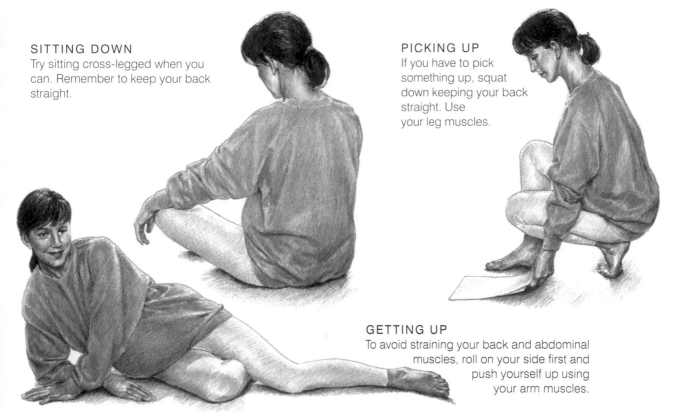

SITTING DOWN
Try sitting cross-legged when you can. Remember to keep your back straight.

PICKING UP
If you have to pick something up, squat down keeping your back straight. Use your leg muscles.

GETTING UP
To avoid straining your back and abdominal muscles, roll on your side first and push yourself up using your arm muscles.

week 32

month   *date*

MON

TUES

WED

THURS

FRI

SAT

SUN

*n*OTES

YOU AND YOUR DEVELOPING BABY

You As your uterus rises and your baby and uterus push up under your diaphragm, the bottom edge of your ribcage may become quite sore.

Baby. Your child is now perfectly formed, although still relatively thin, and his proportions are much as you would expect them to be at birth. If he were born now he would have a very good chance of survival, because his lungs are almost developed. He would, however, need to be placed in an incubator as not enough insulating fat reserves have yet been deposited beneath his skin.

His movements are now very vigorous and may even be quite uncomfortable, especially if his feet get caught under your ribs; sitting up straight will help counteract this. You will probably be aware of him getting hiccups whenever he swallows some amniotic fluid. Each week he will have less and less room to move about and the position he has taken up in the womb, will be checked to see whether he is lying head downwards ready for birth.

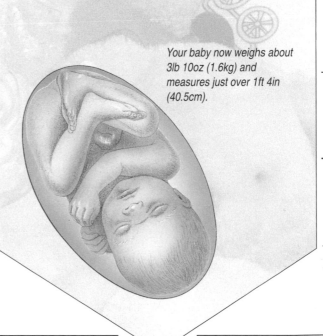

Your baby now weighs about 3lb 10oz (1.6kg) and measures just over 1ft 4in (40.5cm).

Don't forget Begin your childbirth-preparation classes now if you haven't already.

*t*HINKING ABOUT FEEDING

*Y*ou don't have to decide now about how you want to feed your baby, but if you are at all uncertain it is best to start with breast-feeding. It is much more difficult to breast-feed when you have started with bottle-feeding. It is important that you feel positive about the method of feeding you choose. Be honest with yourself and talk over your feelings about feeding; you may have to face up to prejudices about exposing your breasts in front of relatives, for example. Many women worry about the effect breast-feeding might have on their breasts.

Breast-feeding Breast-feeding is certainly best for the health of your baby. Breast milk contains all the nourishment he needs. It is the right temperature and right consistency and being easily digested, is less likely to cause stomach upsets. Breast milk provides antibodies which help to protect your baby against coughs, colds and chest infections; it also helps prevent allergies, such as eczema and asthma.

Breast-feeding is easier and cheaper than bottle-feeding. It is also convenient – your milk is always available, even when travelling. Breast-fed babies are unlikely to get fat. They take as much milk as they need.

Breast-feeding can be emotionally satisfying for the mother. It may also help you regain your figure, due partly to the calories burned up and because the hormones involved in breast-feeding cause contractions of the uterus which help it to return back to its pre-pregnancy size and position.

Many mothers find that breast-feeding is uncomfortable or even painful at first, but this soon settles down.

To avoid cracked nipples, your baby must not simply suck your nipple, but must have as much of the surrounding areola as possible in his mouth as well.

If you feel that breast-feeding could tie you down, remember that you can express your milk for your baby to have in a bottle. It is important to sleep and eat well while feeding and you may have to avoid eating certain foods such as strawberries or spicy things.

The only 'equipment' you will need for breast-feeding are two or three nursing bras (you may want to wear them at night too). They should be easy to open at the front with one hand. You will also need disposable breast pads to soak up leaking milk, or you could use cloth diapers and cut them up into squares.

Bottle-feeding If you do decide to bottle-feed, there is no need to feel guilty. The most important thing is to be relaxed and hold your baby close, no matter how you are feeding him. With bottle-feeding you can see exactly how much milk your baby has taken, and some mothers find this reassuring – it is also an experience that can be shared by the father.

You may, however, find all the sterilizing and preparation required for bottle-feeding hard work, and very time-consuming, at first.

Bottle-feeding is more expensive than breast-feeding. Besides buying the powdered formula milk, you also may need some sterilizing equipment (see below) – but only if you use well water or have any questions about your water supply.

See Week 8
for Buying a Bra

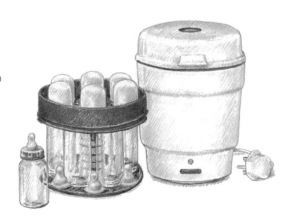

week 33

MON

TUES

WED

THURS

FRI

SAT

SUN

YOU AND YOUR DEVELOPING BABY

You You may find yourself becoming curious about other babies. If you have any friends who have just had a baby, visit them and watch a newborn baby's kicking movements. You may be able to match the movements to those you are feeling in your womb.

If you have difficulty breathing, remember to sit and stand up straight. From around Week 36 this problem should disappear as your baby's head will become 'engaged' (descend into your pelvis).

Baby By now your baby will measure about 1ft 4½in (42cm) and will weigh approximately 4½lb (2kg).

On your notes you will be able to see which way up your baby is 'presenting' – see Understanding your Medical Records, page 88. He is most likely to have settled into a head downwards position. A minority of babies have their bottom downwards, known as 'breech' position. Special delivery techniques may be needed.

The normal position for delivery is head first.

Some babies are in a breech position, presenting bottom first.

*n*OTES

Don't forget Stand up straight at all times and rest for at least an hour a day if you can.

gETTING READY

your mind may be reeling with conflicting emotions; you may worry about whether the baby will be all right, you may be nervous about the birth and at the same time even unsure about whether you really want a baby! The only certain thing is that some time in the next two months your life will totally change and you've got to start preparing for it now. Make preparations now – because those preparations will directly affect everyone's life after the birth.

On the fun side, make the most of your last days of freedom. Visit friends or entertain them. Spoil yourself before there is someone else to look after and rest whenever you can.

On a practical level, begin to get organized. Don't worry about housework, but pack your suitcase for the hospital or gather together the equipment on the list given to you by your mid-

wife for your home birth. Buy or cook some meals for your freezer. Arrange for help at home – a friend, relative – after the birth. And buy enough clothes to keep your baby warm and clean over the first weeks. A baby doesn't need different new clothes for day and night and remember babies grow quickly, so start with the six-month sizes (see below).

Avoid buying synthetic fabrics for the first weeks; especially in summer weather. The baby won't need different clothes for day and night. Remember to buy diapers – either disposable (convenient but expensive), or cloth (cheaper in the long run and ecologically sound, but labor intensive); toiletries (such as baby soap, absorbent cotton, diaper cream) and a book about day-to-day baby care to consult in the future.

See Weeks 28 and 29 for Shopping for Equipment

See Week 36 for Packing your Suitcase

FIRST BABY CLOTHES

4 to 6 stretch suits with snaps around the inside leg so that you don't have to remove the whole outfit for diaper changing.

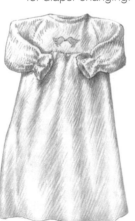

1 or 2 nightgowns: buy long-sleeved, bag-style.

4 undershirts or body shirts which fasten between his legs for extra warmth under a gown or stretch suit.

1 or 2 sweaters and 1 or 2 blanket-sleepers (start out with a bag-style sleeper).

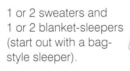

2 pairs mittens in winter.

3 pairs booties or socks: babies' circulation is poor and their feet get cold through not moving around.

1 or 2 knitted hats: babies lose most heat through their head.

Sunhat: to protect a summer baby from the sun.

Bibs, or receiving blankets, to use as bibs in case he throws up milk.

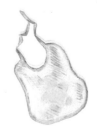

week 34

MON

TUES

WED

THURS

FRI

SAT

SUN

YOU AND YOUR DEVELOPING BABY

You Braxton Hicks contractions usually occur during the last weeks of pregnancy if not before. Although uncomfortable, they are not painful; they are weaker and last less time than labor contractions. If they persist and become stronger, contact your midwife or obstetrician.

Baby Your baby's skin is becoming pinker. He is beginning to be able to differentiate between light and dark. He is also blinking. His lungs are now mature.

During the first stage of labor your cervix (2), normally closed, starts to thin out and to dilate, or open. The contractions of the uterus (1) gradually draw the cervix upwards, over the baby's head.

The dilatation of the cervix is measured in centimeters. At 2-2³/₈in (5-6cm) you are approximately half-dilated. The baby's head is being squeezed lower in the uterus.

At 4in (10cm) the cervix is fully dilated. It has stretched open sufficiently to allow the baby's head to pass through the vagina (3).

*n*OTES

Don't forget Start arranging for friends, relations or paid help to come in and help you after your baby is born.

bREATHING FOR LABOR

Controlled breathing will help you to cope with your contractions by encouraging you to relax your muscles and by distracting your mind and body from any pain you may experience. If you go to prenatal classes you will probably be taught some breathing exercises. It might help you to concentrate if you fix your eyes on an object in the room.

The particular exercises may vary slightly from one hospital, or prenatal class, to another but the principle of breathing for labor remains the same. In some ways, the simpler the breathing the better, because if there are too many different 'levels' to remember you are more likely to become confused during labor, which may make you feel you have lost control. Never worry that you will forget how to breathe properly during labor; your partner will be there to help you.

Aim to slow down your breathing, and learn to concentrate on the outward breath because this is what relaxes you. The inward breath will always take care of itself. Do not hold your breath at any stage, as this increases tension.

See Week 30 for Learning Relaxation

See Week 37 for Onset of Labor

Breathe in through your nose and out through your mouth, concentrating on the outward breath. Make sure you are comfortable and slightly propped up if you are lying on your back.

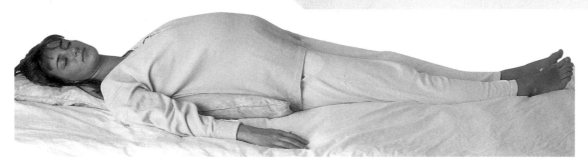

BREATHING TECHNIQUES

Take a breath in through your nose and try to make the air go down to the bottom of your lungs at the base of your ribs. If you are doing this correctly, you will find that your chest moves only a little but your abdomen is pushed out as you breathe in – put one hand on your chest and the other on your stomach to check this.

As you breathe out through your mouth, purse your lips and relax those tense muscles – drop your shoulders and unclench your hands. If you find it difficult to release the tension that is naturally building up, drop your shoulders down and stretch out your hands to unclench your tensed muscles. Breathe a sigh of relief at the end of the contraction.

If you become breathless during your exercises, you are breathing too fast – make a conscious effort to slow down. If you become dizzy, it means that you are breathing in too strongly (hyperventilating): cup your hands tightly round your mouth and breathe normally in and out several times until you feel better. Then continue on with the exercises, making the 'out' breath stronger.

week 35

MON

TUES

WED

THURS

FRI

SAT

SUN

*n*OTES

YOU AND YOUR DEVELOPING BABY

You Don't stand or sit in one position for too long; not only may your ankles swell, but your body may become increasingly immobile. Rest as much of the day as you can.
Baby Your baby is rapidly losing his wrinkled appearance and becoming plumper. Between now and birth more fat will be deposited all over his body, mainly around the shoulders.

The hair on his head is growing and his soft toe- and fingernails have grown almost to the ends of his fingers and toes.

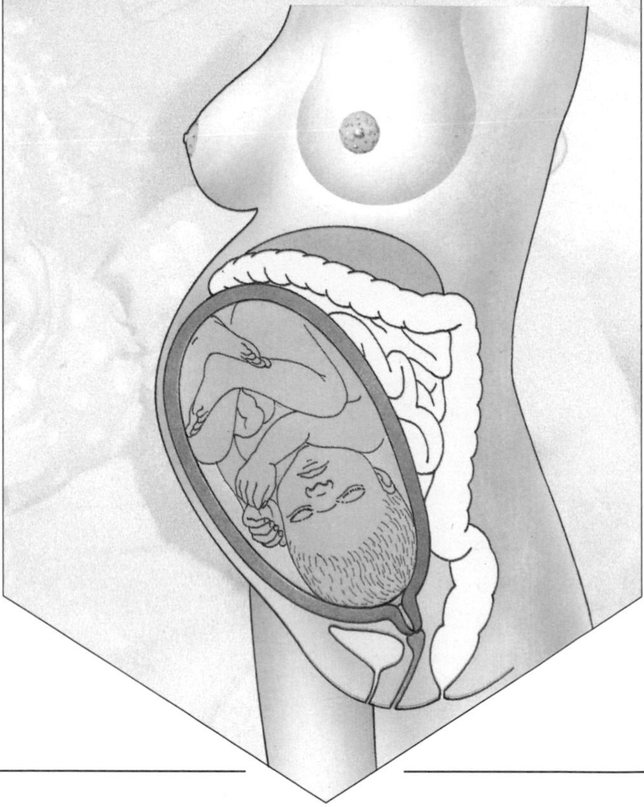

Don't forget If you plan to breast-feed your baby, buy three nursing bras.

*l*abor is usually painful, to a greater or lesser degree, therefore it's a good idea to know what kinds of pain relief are readily available so you can think about, and discuss them before it all starts. However, you should always be prepared to be flexible about any decisions you make. Whatever you imagine your labor will be like, it is bound to be different. Remember that it is not a sin to change your mind. Let your doctor or midwife advise you.

HAVING AN EPIDURAL

For most women an epidural gives complete pain relief and for a long or very painful labor it may be an ideal solution. It is a special type of local anaesthetic that works by blocking the nerves which carry the feelings of pain from your uterus, cervix and vagina to your brain. It can even be used for a cesarean section, allowing the mother to remain conscious for the birth.

The disadvantage of an epidural is that you may not be able to move about, or even change position, without help. Since you probably won't be able to feel your contractions either, you may not feel the urge to push and will have to be told when to

do so. This may mean it takes longer to push your baby out or that the baby has to be delivered by forceps.

If you know in advance that you want an epidural it is a good idea to ask as soon as you get into the labour room as the anaesthetist may be in demand around the hospital.

Having an epidural is not painful, as your back is numbed before it is given. You lie curled up on your side on the edge of the bed and a needle is injected between the bones of your spine. A plastic tube is threaded down the needle into a place outside the nerves of the spinal cord. The needle is then removed and the

tube is held in place on your back by sticky tape. The anesthetic is injected down the tube and takes about fifteen minutes to work.

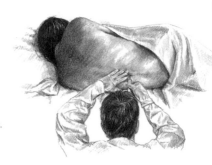

See Week 34 for Breathing for Labor

See Week 40 for The Birth

OTHER FORMS OF PAIN RELIEF

General anesthesia
In the past, women in labor were routinely given general anesthetics but this practice is seldom used today because of complications. The use of analgesics (drugs which relieve or diminish the intensity of pain but do not cause unconsciousness) and local anesthetics (such as epidurals) is much more common. Occasionally, however, certain

mild gases such as nitrous oxide, which you breath in through a face mask that covers your mouth and nose, are used during labor. Though they do not put you to sleep, these can make it very difficult to concentrate on using other pain relief techniques, such as breathing and relaxation.
Meperidine and alphaprodine
Meperidine and alphaprodine are the most widely used injected drugs. You may find they help

with the pain but injected drugs can make you feel, or even be, sick. Or they may make you so sleepy that you can't push when you need to.

Hypnosis, acupuncture and aromatherapy massage techniques are other means of pain relief. You will need to practise these methods beforehand and be prepared to opt for something stronger if they don't work.

week 36

MON

_____

TUES

_____

WED

_____

THURS

_____

FRI

_____

SAT

_____

SUN

_____

*n*OTES

YOU AND YOUR DEVELOPING BABY

You The top of your uterus has reached just below your breastbone. This will make breathing uncomfortable and may also give you a jabbing pain in your ribcage.

If this is your first baby, 'lightening' may occur sometime during the next few weeks. This is when your baby's head 'engages', or drops into your pelvis, which indicates that he can pass through your pelvic cavity without difficulty. With a second or subsequent pregnancy, lightening may not occur until just before labor begins. Prenatal visits are weekly from now on.

Baby All your baby's organs are now almost mature and if he is born he has a ninety per cent chance of survival.

Your baby's head has probably dropped into your pelvis.

Don't forget Pack your suitcases now.

*p*ACKING YOUR SUITCASE

*d*epending on the type of birth you have had and the policy of your hospital or birthing center, you could be home as soon as eight to 24-hours after giving birth. As you probably won't know beforehand, take the bare minimum – your partner or visiting family and friends can always bring in anything you have forgotten.

Remember to pack your bags several weeks before your due date (especially if you are having twins) so you don't have to worry about anything once you have gone into labor except getting to the hospital.

You might also think it is worth packing a suitcase for your partner to bring in when it is time for you to come home. This should contain a loose outfit for you as your figure won't be back to its original shape – it should also be front-opening if you are breast-feeding. The baby's home coming clothes and blanket or shawl can be placed in the car safety seat. Make sure the proper restraints are fitted ready for the trip home. In winter, make sure the house is warm for your homecoming.

See Week 33 for First Baby Clothes

See Week 38 for Fathers in Labor

FOR THE LABOR

- Your insurance card or number.
- Ice packs for backache.
- A washcloth and an atomizer to cool you down.
- Warm socks (you may get cold during labor).
- Chapstick or lip balm.
- High-energy snacks (nuts, raisins, candy bars) to sustain your partner during a long labor.
- Portable CD or tape player and favorite music if they will help you relax and if they are allowed in the labor room.
- Toiletries such as toothbrush, toothpaste, hairbrush or comb, and elastic to tie back long hair.
- A hand mirror (if you want to watch the birth).
- Crosswords, playing cards.
- Camera (if you want your partner to photograph the birth).
- Lots of change for pay phone, vending machines.
- If you have taken a Lamaze class, you may also want to bring such things as tennis balls, lollipops, a watch with a second hand to time contractions, or even a favorite picture or photograph to focus on during labor.

FOR AFTERWARDS

- 2 extra front-opening nightgowns.
- Slippers and a robe.
- Six pairs of underpants.
- Address book, birth announcements, stamps and pen.
- Earplugs and eyeshades to help you sleep.
- Other toiletries such as shampoo, soap, deodorant, face creams and make-up.
- Favorite book or magazine to read.
- 2 nursing bras; breast pads.
- Drinks for you and your guests, such as sparkling cider or spring water.
- Diapers and baby clothes – allow for a few changes.
- One pacifier.

week 37

month   *date*

MON

TUES

WED

THURS

FRI

SAT

SUN

YOU AND YOUR DEVELOPING BABY

Your baby could be born any day from now until the end of Week 42. The average duration of a twin pregnancy is only 37 weeks so prepare yourself now if they haven't yet appeared. Second, third and fourth babies are also more often early than late.

● If you have a family, finalize all arrangements for your children to be cared for while you're away.

● Make sure you know where your partner is at all times – ask him to leave all his telephone numbers with you.

● Keep your car filled with gas and put a blanket in the back for comfort on the trip to the hospital. If you plan to go by taxi, keep the telephone numbers of at least two 24-hour taxi companies by your phone and some money for the fare.

● Get your baby's room, layette and crib ready.

Important telephone numbers	
Partner at work:	Neighbors:
Doctor's office:	Your parents:
Midwife/Hospital:	Partner's parents:
School number:	Ambulance:
	Taxi:

*n*OTES

Don't forget If you're at all worried, call your doctor or midwife: better to be safe than sorry.

ONSET OF LABOR

even though you may not believe this now, you will probably know when you are in labor. There's no point losing sleep worrying over whether tonight is going to be the night, although you probably will have the odd night of anxiety, everyone does. But no one has ever had a baby in their sleep. You'll be woken up if anything is about to happen, and, if it's not, you need to get all the rest you can to keep you fit for the actual day.

The most obvious 'signs' to watch out for are described below and one or more of them will indicate that labor has started or it will soon. Should you experience any of the three sensations listed below, or if you are at any time worried, call your doctor (or midwife, if you're having an out-of-hospital birth) and tell them. Don't worry that you might be raising a false alarm: doctors are used to this. Keep your blood sugar levels up with light snacks.

See Week 36 for Packing Your Suitcase

Contractions The muscles of your womb will start to tighten up and will feel rather like bad period pains or a fist clenching. This is a labor contraction and it will feel stronger and more pronounced than Braxton Hicks contractions.

Time the spaces between your contractions and when they are coming about every ten minutes, or earlier if you can't cope any longer, telephone the doctor (or your midwife if you are having an out-of-hospital birth). Early in labor, you can safely drink liquids.

With a second or subsequent baby, contractions are likely to remain quite mild and infrequent until labor is advanced. They can then suddenly change to long, strong contractions, so don't delay calling the doctor.

A 'show' This is when the plug of mucus at the cervix (neck of the uterus) comes away as the uterus starts to open. You may notice a small discharge of blood-streaked jelly. Telephone the doctor, tell her that you have had a 'show', and they will tell you what to do.

Rupturing of the membranes This is when the bag of amniotic fluid in which your baby is floating breaks and the amniotic fluid starts to come out. It is known as 'the waters breaking'. This usually happens towards the end of the first stage of labor but may happen at the onset of labor or several days before. You'll notice either a small leak or a gush of warm fluid escaping from your vagina. It may feel like a period starting and it may be accompanied by some bleeding. Telephone the doctor at once.

The sticky plug of mucus (1) that seals the cervical canal (2) during pregnancy is dislodged once the cervix (3) begins to dilate. The slightly blood-stained, jelly-like discharge is known as 'the show' when it is released. It may not mean that labor has started, although it indicates that your cervix is opening a little. It may not be dislodged until labor is well under way.

TELEPHONE THE HOSPITAL IMMEDIATELY IF . . .

- Your waters break.
- You have any bleeding. If you are bleeding heavily, rest with your feet up until an ambulance arrives.
- Your contractions are coming more frequently than every ten minutes or are painful.

Remember to allow for the time it will take to get to the hospital, so don't delay telephoning the doctor for too long.

week 38

month   *date*

MON

TUES

WED

THURS

FRI

SAT

SUN

YOU AND YOUR DEVELOPING BABY

You You may feel bulky and a little bored with your pregnancy by now, or may be getting depressed about having your baby. Don't be alarmed by any shooting pains in your groin and down your legs – it probably means that your baby's head has engaged and is moving against your pelvic floor muscles or resting on a nerve. On the whole, however, he is probably moving about less.

Baby The fine lanugo hair covering your baby's body will begin to disappear, although some may remain on his shoulders and in the creases of his body.

Your baby may be putting on up to 1oz (28g) a day in weight, but your weight will probably remain steady from now on.

*n*OTES

Don't forget Look at these pages with your partner.

*f*ATHERS IN LABOR

*l*abor is one of the hardest, most emotional and most painful experiences you will go through together. Labor itself, and the way you will feel during it, are totally unpredictable for both of you. At worst you will snap at your partner, tell him you hate him being there, scream when he touches you – and shout at him to shut up when he asks you how he can help. At some stage you are bound to tell him you'll never have another child, and – at that moment – you will mean it! To prepare your partner for your (and his) unpredictability, ask him to read this:

Fathers, be prepared for all of this and don't hold it against your partner. Instead, support her and tell her she is being very brave – she is! Your presence will be invaluable if you can try to second-guess what she wants. Make yourself invisible when she doesn't need you.

Respect your partner's wishes and allow that she may change her mind about pain relief or anything else. You're not experiencing the birth – she is. If she wants an epidural having talked about 'natural birth', that's fine. Give comfort in any way you can. Have an open mind and listen to the doctor's advice.

See Week 24 for The Father's Role

See Week 36 for Packing Your Suitcase

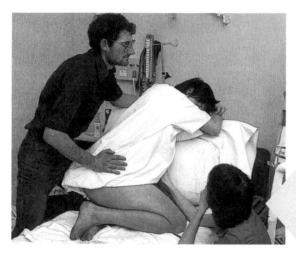

Make sure she is well supported and relaxed at all times. During labor see that she has everything she needs, and stroke or massage her if it helps. But don't feel rejected if she wants to be left alone.

TIPS FOR LABOR PARTNERS

- Your role will begin the moment your partner starts labor. It is especially important *before* you get to the hospital, when there is no one else around. Work with her through her relaxation and breathing techniques now, before labor proper.
- Labor can take any shape or form so keep an open mind and always remember that there is no 'right' or 'wrong'
- No matter how useless you may feel at some points

during labor, be reassured that your very presence is supportive.
- During her contractions you can 'breathe' with her, especially if you see she's getting mixed up and needs reinforcement. In the early stages, you can walk around with her and let her lean against you.
- Always be relaxed yourself. It may be enough for you just to sit in the corner of the room reading. Have something to

eat to keep your strength up. Ask the nurse-midwife if there is anything you can do.
- During labor if your partner says she is in pain, agree with her. Don't pretend the pain isn't there. Instead, congratulate her on how well she is doing.
- Giving birth is a highly emotional state. Don't be surprised if your partner gets upset and if you, too, find yourself slightly overwhelmed and disturbed emotionally.

week 39

month   *date*

MON

TUES

WED

THURS

FRI

SAT

SUN

*n*OTES

YOU AND YOUR DEVELOPING BABY

You If this is your first baby, your womb will now be approximately three fingers below your breastbone – as in Week 34 – if lightening has occurred.

You will probably be feeling quite exhausted by now and may just want to stay at home with your feet up. Do just that – rest is essential. Let your partner know how you are feeling at all times.

Baby Your baby's intestine is filled with meconium, a sticky, dark greenish-black substance made up of the excretions from his alimentary glands mixed with bile pigment, lanugo and cells from the bowel wall. This will be his first bowel movement, which will be passed during the first two days of his life, and possibly also during labor, so don't get a shock when you see it.

Don't forget You can cry if you feel like it – don't be ashamed.

pOSITIONS IN LABOR

$t$oday many doctors and midwives advocate being in an upright position (standing or squatting) during labor. No matter which birthing position you choose, it is important for you to feel comfortable and to give your baby as much room as possible.

For an active birth, during which you stand, sit, kneel, rock, walk about or squat, it is important that you discuss your views with your doctor well in advance (see Week 9); you may have to find a hospital that has the facilities for women to be active during labor, such as the newer birthing chairs. Bear in mind that an active birth means you need a support partner (or two). It also means you can't have an epidural.

It is important that you trust the medical staff who are delivering your baby and cooperate with them. Don't be upset if you end up propped up on a hospital bed with a fetal monitor strapped to your abdomen or an intravenous drip in your arm or if you have a Caesarean. The richness of your labor experience won't be lessened by any of these things, it will just be different.

See Week 31 for Good Posture

See Week 9 for Prenatal Care

ACTIVE BIRTH? PROS AND CONS

- If you are left to find the position that suits you, your pain may be reduced.
- Squatting or kneeling puts pelvic organs in the best position to deliver your baby.
- In an upright position your uterus won't press on the artery leading to the heart, which may give your baby a better chance of getting his oxygen supply.
- Being upright can promote stronger contractions in the first stage. This may lessen the need for forceps or episiotomy.
- If you are upright you have the force of gravity on your side.
- An upright position allows for spontaneous delivery of the placenta.
- Propped up on a bed may be more restful for you.
- If you're on a bed it's easier for the doctor and midwife to examine you.

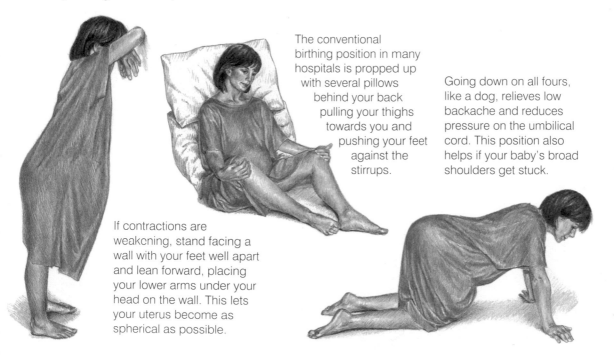

The conventional birthing position in many hospitals is propped up with several pillows behind your back pulling your thighs towards you and pushing your feet against the stirrups.

Going down on all fours, like a dog, relieves low backache and reduces pressure on the umbilical cord. This position also helps if your baby's broad shoulders get stuck.

If contractions are weakening, stand facing a wall with your feet well apart and lean forward, placing your lower arms under your head on the wall. This lets your uterus become as spherical as possible.

week 40

month   *date*

MON

TUES

WED

THURS

FRI

SAT

SUN

YOU AND YOUR DEVELOPING BABY

You You may be nervous as the expected date of delivery approaches. However, only five per cent of babies arrive on time.

Baby His skin is soft and smooth and most of the lanugo has disappeared. His body is completely covered with vernix.

Don't get a shock when you see him for the first time. He may be blue in color, some of his head and body will still be covered with white, cheesy-looking vernix, and may also be smeared with your blood. He will be wet and slippery, his hair will have stuck to his face and he will probably be pulling an angry face just before taking his first breath: in addition, his head may still have a strange shape after the passage down the birth canal. You won't be looking that great either!

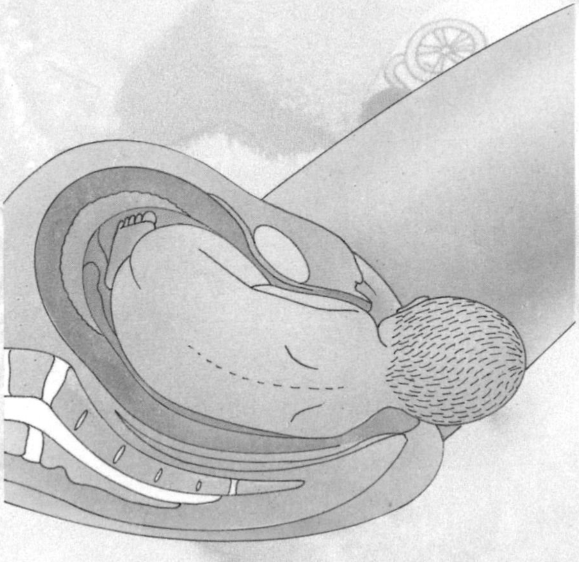

Your fully developed baby is soon to leave your womb.

Don't forget Give up all preconceptions. Keep an open mind throughout the birth.

*n*OTES

*Y*ou will have lived through your baby's birth countless times in your mind, but this time it will be for real. It is unlikely to be as you have imagined and, realistically, it may well be worse. Remember that whatever pain you are going through will end. There are drugs to help you through it, should you want them. On the day everyone will be on your side, so let them help you. But remember that labor is something you are doing.

Don't be disappointed if you can't have the 'natural' birth you planned for. All births are natural and there is certainly nothing artificial about your baby. Equally, don't feel bad if the 'bonding' with your baby isn't immediate; it may take some time to get to know each other.

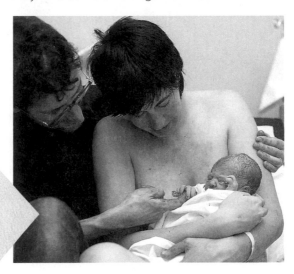

There is no such thing as the perfect birth. Nor is there such a thing as failure in labor, as there is no standard to be achieved. Each labor is highly individual and you should be prepared to work with whatever your own labor brings.

The first stage The first stage is when your cervix, which is usually closed, starts to dilate or open up. Your contractions, caused by the muscles of the womb shrinking, will slowly open up your cervix until it is about 10cm (4in) wide and ready to let your baby through.

Concentrate on the relaxation and breathing you learned as best you can. Take each contraction at a time and don't let anyone or anything interfere with them. Don't feel you need to be polite during a contraction; no one expects you to.

Your contractions will gradually become stronger and more painful and you may start feeling you want to push (this is known as the 'transition' stage). To stop yourself pushing, lift your head and blow out in little puffs of air, or pant, making sure that your mouth, legs and pelvic floor are completely relaxed.

The second stage The second stage of labor is when your baby is born. Your cervix should be fully dilated before you start pushing. Keep your chin tucked well down and your mouth closed as you give long, slow pushes.

The third stage The third stage is the delivery of the placenta. This stage is usually very quick and easy. As your baby is born, you'll probably be given an injection in your thigh to help your womb contract. A final contraction will then push out the placenta. Any necessary stitching up will be done next. This is your first opportunity to see and hold your new baby.

INDUCTION
There are many reasons why your labor might have to be started artificially. It could be that you have high blood pressure or diabetes, or your baby is some weeks late. It could be that you have no contractions.

One method of induction is known as ARM (artificial rupture of the membranes). Your membranes are pierced, allowing some of the amniotic fluid to escape. By altering the pressure in your womb this causes labor to start. Another method is by dripping a synthetic hormone directly into your bloodstream.

See Week 34 for Dilatation of the Cervix

See Week 35 for Pain Relief

See Week 37 for Onset of Labor

See Week 39 for Positions in Labor

See page 86 for After the Birth

*a*FTER THE BIRTH

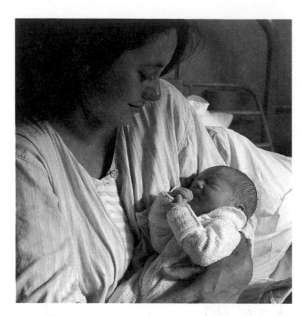

*n*o matter what kind of birth you had, or how you are feeling about your new baby, life may suddenly seem a bit of an anticlimax after the experiences you have been through. Parts of your body may hurt and although you may be one of the lucky mothers who love their new baby from the moment he appears, you are just as likely to look at him in amazement and wonder where he came from and what you are expected to do with him.

If you are in a hospital, this may be the only time you have in which you can concentrate exclusively on yourself and your baby without domestic responsibilities, so take advantage of it. Use your stay to get to know your baby and to learn how to care for him with the help of the hospital staff. Spend some time on yourself too: a manicure or writing a thank you – or even a little note to yourself on how you feel now pregnancy is over – and catch up on some much-needed sleep. You have a period of great adjustment ahead of you.

If you've had a home birth, you must delegate as much as possible to your partner, friends and family. Your midwife should be on-call to answer questions. She will be able to advise you on how to look after yourself and your baby. Over the next ten days she, or one

of her colleagues, will no doubt visit you. Don't hesitate to ask her for advice about anything.

Getting to know your baby
In many hospitals today you can request 'full rooming-in,' which means that the baby can stay with you in your room throughout the day, except for visiting hours, and all night. Your hospital may also offer a modified rooming-in option whereby you can have your baby with you in your hospital room during the daytime, except for visiting hours. At night the baby goes back to the nursery and is brought to you either on demand or at regular designated intervals for feedings. Don't feel guilty if you're tired and you don't choose full rooming-in. You're wise to realize that you'll need your rest for the days ahead.

Whatever you do though, be sure to take advantage of the postpartum care staff. They are there to help and can offer you invaluable practical guidance and support.

The hospital routine
The doctors usually do their rounds in the morning and will check on you and the baby; the afternoons are generally more restful and there is usually a period of enforced quiet – use it! Although you may want to share the excitement of your baby with all your friends and family, bear in mind that visitors can be very tiring, especially in the first few days. It is also important to spend some time alone with your partner.

Looking after yourself
If you have had an exhausting labor, you can usually ask the hospital staff to look after your baby for the first night so that you can catch up on lost sleep. Nobody will think the worse of you for this; you will be woken if he needs feeding. On the other hand your emotional 'high' may stop you from sleeping during the first night after delivery – you may still be too excited, or may find yourself reliving the birth every time you close your eyes.

The physical strain of labor may make you ache severely and it may be a great effort to drag yourself to the bathroom for the first day or so. If you had an episiotomy, your stitches may give you pain, especially when you sit down. Don't be afraid to ask for painkillers: they will help you to get through the first days.

You may suffer from constipation for a few days after the birth. This can be aggravated if you are worried about your stitches bursting (which they will not). Drink plenty of liquid, and eat fresh fruit and vegetables and 'high-fiber' cereals to ensure that the first bowel movement is soft enough to pass without too much difficulty. If necessary your doctor will suggest some medication.

You will find you bleed quite heavily for a few days after the birth and that you continue to have a brown discharge for several weeks after that. This discharge is called lochia. Use sanitary napkins and not internal tampons.

Breast-feeding
Your breasts will feel tender and become 'engorged', around the third or fourth day when the milk first comes in. Your nipples may also become sore when your baby first begins to suck. But persevere – all these initial problems will be overcome.

Postpartum blues
You may well feel a bit depressed a few days after your baby is born. The level of hormones present in your bloodstream during pregnancy quickly decreases after the birth and your body has to adjust accordingly.

Whatever happens during the first few weeks, don't worry or be discouraged when things go wrong. Remind yourself what an emotional and tiring experience you've been through. The next wonder of nature is that in a few months you'll have forgotten almost all of it, as you settle into your life as a mother. You'll have just one beautiful souvenir – your baby.

POSTPARTUM EXERCISES

Start postpartum exercises as soon after the birth as you feel able – while you are still in the hospital. Strenuous exercises, such as lying on your back and either lifting both legs up and then lowering them, or 'bicycling' with both legs raised, should not be done for at least six weeks after delivery.

Most of the postpartum exercises can be done in bed or, later on, lying on the floor. Do each one six times, relaxing after each. Continue them for at least six weeks after the birth.

Days 1 and 2 after birth
1 Lie on your back with your legs straight and slightly apart. Bend and stretch your ankles, then your toes, then circle your feet in both directions.

2 Lie on your back with your knees bent and your feet resting on the bed or floor. Tighten your buttock muscles and pull in your abdomen so that your back is pressed against the bed. Hold for six, then relax.

Day 3 after the birth
Introduce the following to the above exercises:

3 Practice your pelvic floor exercise (see Week 15) lying flat on your back on your bed with your knees bent.

Day 4 after the birth
Introduce the following:

4 Lie with your right knee bent and your right foot on the bed and your left leg straight with the foot flexed. Slide the heel of your left leg up and down the bed, keeping your leg straight and using only your waist muscles. Change legs.

5 Lie with your knees bent and your feet on the bed. Pull in your abdominal muscles and reach across your body to place one hand on the opposite side of the bed at hip level. Return that hand to its starting position and do the same with the other hand.

*a*t some point you may want to take a look at your medical records. Because doctors and hospitals are often reluctant to provide access to medical records, you may be asked to put your request in writing first and go in person to the hospital's medical records department. Call the health care provider whose records you wish to see and ask what procedure you should follow. (Bear in mind that a patient's medical record is a legal document and not his or her property.) Most of the abbreviations that you will see on your prenatal record are explained below. If there is anything that you do not understand, or if you simply can't read the midwife's or the consultant's writing, ask for it to be explained.

PRE-NATAL RECORD

INVESTIGATIONS	DATE	RESULTS	DRUGS	FIRST EXAMINATION 10·4·92		α FETOPROTEIN	
A.B.O. Blood Group		A		Height	1·70	SERUM:–	
Rhesus Blood Group		positive		Breasts	NAD	Date	
Antibodies	10/4/92.	Neg		Heart	knew	OTHER TESTS	
WR/KAHN		Neg		Lungs	clear		
RUBELLA ANTIBODIES		Immune	ALLERGIES	Varicose Veins	No		
AUSTRALIA ANTIGEN		Neg		Pelvis			
Cx SMEAR				⬡ 14/40. Sugar			

DATE	WEEKS	UTERINE SIZE	URINE ALB. SUGAR	B.P.	WEIGHT. Kg	PRESENTA-TION AND POSITION	RELATION OF P.P. TO BRIM	F.H.	EDEMA	Hb	NEXT VISIT	SIG.	COMM
10/4/92	14+4/7	14	NAD	120/70	86kg	–	–	FHH	nil	88	level II	Barton	Not
24.7.92	19+2	= 20/40	NAD	110/70	90kg				First	11·3		EAB	2
26.6.92	26	=	nor.	100/55		U.S.							2C
24/7/92	29	30cm	Sug	120/70	94	661C	NE	FH	81	Hb AB	60CH 95	9A	for B
29/7/92	29+6	BSS	3-7 mmol			6-4 mmol		J.O mmol			FHH		
5.8.92	31	30cm	nil nil	110/60	93	Breech		H				tra	
20.8.92	33	32cm	nil nil	110/60	94	Breech	NE	H				tra	
17.9.92	37	≡	– –	110/60	95	C	NE	FHH slight	–	2/52.	Cl	
25/9/92	38	38 cm	NAD	110/60	98	C	4/5	FHHr nil.		②	Cl	
28.9.92	38+	≡		110/70.		C	4/5	FHH nil			Cl	Abd
5.10.92	39+	≡	NAD	120/70.		C	4/5	FHH		②	Cl	
9.10.92	T+8	40cm	NAD	120/80	100	C	4/5	H	u	①	9A	PV
16-10.92	T+8	–	tr pr	100/60	995	C	3/5	TM		102 Sug/TM		
												PLANNE
												● 48 HC
												● 5 DA
												● 9 DA
												● OTHE

Date
The date of your prenatal visit.

Weeks
The length of your pregnancy in weeks, from the first day of your last menstrual period.

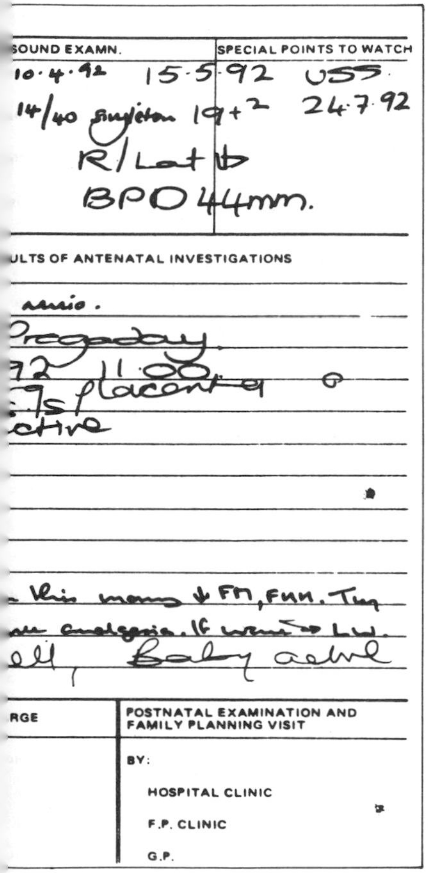

Urine Alb. Sugar
This shows the result of your urine tests for protein and sugar. 'Tr' or '+' means a trace (or quantity) has been found; 'Alb' stands for albumin, one of the proteins that could be found in your urine. 'Ketones' means you are low in energy. 'NAD', 'Nil', or a dash all mean nothing abnormal.

B.P.
Blood Pressure. This should stay at about the same level throughout pregnancy. If it goes up it can be dangerous for you and your baby.

Weight
This is your weight in pounds.

Presentation and position
This shows which way up your baby is lying or 'presenting'. 'Vx' means vertex; 'C' or 'ceph' means cephalic. Both words literally mean the top of the head and show that your baby has settled into a head downwards position and is ready to be born head first. 'Breech' means that your baby has his bottom downwards. 'PP' means presenting part – the bit of your baby that is coming first.

Up to about Week 36 your baby moves about a lot and then usually settles down. You may find your doctor or midwife only start filling in this column then.

Uterine size/Height of fundus
This is the distance in centimeters from your pelvis to the top of your womb, i.e. the height of your fundus. The figure should be roughly the same as that in the 'Weeks' column.

Relation of PP to Brim
This is where your baby's head (the 'presenting part') is situated in relation to the brim of your pelvis. 'E' or 'Eng' means engaged. The engaging of your baby's head is expressed in fifths.

So 5/5ths means he is beginning to engage, 4/5ths means he has dropped further down and so on. 'NE' means not engaged.

Abbreviations are also used to describe the way your baby is lying in your abdomen. The 'O' stands for occiput (the crown of your baby's head); the 'R' and 'L' for whether the baby is on the right or left side of your body and the 'A' and 'P' for whether your baby's back is facing to the front (anterior) or to the back (posterior) of your body.

FH
'FHH', or 'H', or a check mark means fetal heart heard. 'FHNH' is fetal heart not heard. 'FMF' is fetal movements felt.

Edema
This is the swelling, usually of your hands, feet and ankles (see Week 26) which can lead to further problems; '+' means you have edema and each further '+' denotes the degree of swelling.

Hb
'Hb' stands for hemoglobin. This is tested in your blood to see whether you are anemic. 'Fe' means that iron has been prescribed.

Next visit
The approximate date of your next visit is written in this column. 4/52 means in four week's time, 1/52 means in one week's time and so on.

Sig.
The doctor will initial this box after he has finished giving you your checkup.

(handwritten form)

SOUND EXAMN.	SPECIAL POINTS TO WATCH
10·4·92 15·5·92	USS.
14/40 *anytion* 19+²	24·7·92

R/Lat ↓
BPO 44mm.

RESULTS OF ANTENATAL INVESTIGATIONS

amio.
Pregaday.
72 11.00
9s placenta O
active

this means ↓ FM, FMM. They are analgesic. If want to L.W.
oll, Baby achve

RGE	POSTNATAL EXAMINATION AND FAMILY PLANNING VISIT
	BY:
	HOSPITAL CLINIC
	F.P. CLINIC
	G.P.

gLOSSARY

Afterbirth
See Placenta

Amniocentesis
A test sometimes performed during pregnancy which is used to detect chromosomal disorders such as Down's syndrome (see Week 17).

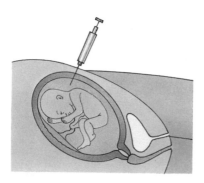

Amniotic sac
Inside your uterus your baby is floating in an oval bag formed of two thin tissues (membranes) called the amniotic sac. It is filled with waters (amniotic fluid) which cushion the baby from any knocks and jolts during pregnancy. Before or during labor, the membranes will break and the amniotic fluid will leak out. This is called 'breaking the waters' (see Week 37).

Analgesia
An analgesic is a pain-easing agent which does not cause unconsciousness. The analgesics that are most commonly used in labor are meperidine and alphaprodine which are given by injection (see Week 35).

Braxton Hicks contractions
These are thought to be the uterus's way of preparing for the contractions of labor (see Contractions). They occur every twenty minutes throughout pregnancy, although you may only notice them during the last few weeks. They feel like a painless but uncomfortable hardening across the stomach (see Week 23).

Breech presentation
Most babies are born head first, that is the head is the presenting part. A baby in a breech presentation means that his bottom is presenting and he will come out bottom (or, in rare cases, legs) first. It is not a particularly common phenomenon; only about four in every hundred babies are breech.

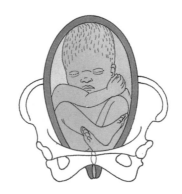

Cesarean section
This is when your baby is delivered by cutting through your abdomen into your womb. Your baby, membranes and placenta are lifted out and you are sewn up. The operation takes place either under general or epidural anaesthetic (so you can be awake during the delivery) and takes about 40 minutes. If your doctor or midwife considers that a vaginal delivery would be dangerous or impossible for you, you may have a planned ('elective') cesarean, in which case you can help to choose your date of delivery. The operation is sometimes carried out in an emergency, for example, during a labor if the baby appears distressed.

Cervix
This is the neck of your uterus, the part which looks like the narrow part of the pear (see Uterus). It is 1in (2.5cm) long and when you are not pregnant remains almost completely closed with just a small opening through which blood passes during your monthly period. During labor, muscular contractions gradually open up the cervix more and more until it is about 4in (10cm) wide, so that your baby can pass through it.

Contractions
Regular tightening of the muscles of the uterus. During labor these become more forceful and will push your baby down the birth canal.

EDC/EDD
Expected date of confinement or expected date of delivery.

Embryo
The embryo is the fertilized egg in the early stages of pregnancy. As it grows it becomes known as a 'fetus', usually from Week 7.

Engaged
About Week 36 in a first pregnancy (later for subsequent pregnancies), your baby's head will drop down into your pelvis so

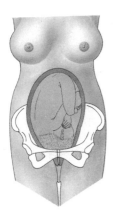

the widest part of his head is through your pelvic brim. Also known as 'lightening'.

Epidural
An anaesthetic used in labor to relieve your pain while leaving you fully conscious. It is done by an injection into the fluid surrounding your spinal cord (see Week 35).

Episiotomy
An incision made in your perineum if necessary just before your baby is born in order to enlarge the exit for him and to prevent you tearing.

Fallopian tubes
Two narrow tubes about 4in (10cm) long which lead from your ovaries to your uterus.

Fetus
See Embryo

Fundus
The top of your uterus (see Week 20).

Gestation
The period from conception to birth (i.e. 40 weeks).

Hormones
Chemicals produced by the body to perform functions in particular to do with growth and reproduction. They have a variety of effects during pregnancy.

Induction
Any process which starts labor artificially (see Week 40).

Labor
The process of childbirth.

Lanugo
A growth of fine hair which will appear all over your baby's body as a protection during pregnancy (see Week 16).

Lightening
See Engaged.

Membranes
See Amniotic sac.

Miscarriage
The loss of a baby before twenty-eight weeks' gestation. The risk of miscarriage is highest in the first twelve weeks of pregnancy.

Mucus
See Plug of mucus.

Ovaries
There are two ovaries (female sex glands) in your body, each of which is about the size of a large almond. Every month one of them expels an egg, or ovum, which weaves its way down the fallopian tube in search of male sperm on the way up from the vagina.

Perineum
The area between your vagina and anus.

Placenta
An organ grown solely to nourish your baby and to excrete his waste products. It is a more or less circular piece of tissue, attached on the one side to your uterus and on the other to your baby via his umbilical cord. The placenta works like a sieve, allowing oxygen, food and protective antibodies to be passed from you to your baby, but in the same way toxic substances can be filtered through as well. The placenta also passes your baby's waste products to you for disposal. The placenta, or 'afterbirth', is expelled through the vagina shortly after your baby is born in what is known as the third stage of labor.

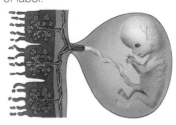

Plug of mucus
Placed in the cervix, like a cork in the neck of a bottle, the plug of mucus seals off the contents of your uterus from outside

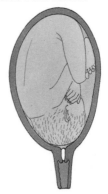

interference and protects your baby from infection. The plug comes out in order for the waters to break (see Week 37).

Prenatal
Before birth.

Primagravida
A woman pregnant for the first time. An 'elderly primagravida', in medical terms, is anyone over the age of twenty-five having a first baby.

Quickening
The first movements of your baby inside the uterus.

Rubella
Another name for German measles (see Week 2).

Stillbirth
The delivery of a baby who has already died in the uterus after twenty-eight weeks of pregnancy.

Trimester
Pregnancy is divided into three trimesters (literally thirds of pregnancy). The first is the first thirteen weeks of pregnancy, the second lasts from Week 14 to Week 27 and the third is from Week 28 until delivery (see Week 4).

Ultrasound
A highly sophisticated instrument which uses soundwaves to show the development of the baby in your uterus (see Week 16).

Umbilical cord
This is the link between you (your placenta) and your baby. Blood circulates through the cord, carrying oxygen and food to your baby and removing waste. The cord measures about 2ft (60cm). (See also Placenta.)

Uterus
Before impregnation your uterus (womb) is about the same shape and size as a small, upsidedown pear, weighs about 2oz (55g) and is hollow with a thick muscular wall. At the top it is joined on either side to the fallopian tubes; the other narrow end is called the cervix.

When you become pregnant the fertilized egg embeds itself in the lining of the uterus and your unborn baby remains in there until the end of your pregnancy. By the time your baby is fully formed, the uterus is a powerful 2lb (0.9kg) muscle-mass capable of pushing your baby out.

Vagina
Your vagina is a tube of muscle about 3-4in (8-10cm) long which leads from your cervix to your vulva, your external sexual organ. The vagina forms the birth canal during labor.

Womb
See Uterus.

When writing for information please enclose a stamped addressed envelope.

PRENATAL CARE AND BIRTH
American Academy of Bradley Childbirth Method
P.O. Box 5224
Sherman Oaks, CA 91413
800-788-6662 (toll-free outside CA)
800-42-BIRTH (toll-free CA only)
Information and referrals to prenatal classes emphasizing the Bradley/Dick-Read childbirth method

American College of Nurse Midwives
818 Connecticut Ave., N.W.
Washington, D.C.
Suite 900
Washington, D.C. 20006
202-728-9860
National directory of nurse-midwife practices ($6.95, incl. postage)

American Society of Psychoprophylaxis in Obstetrics (ASPO/LAMAZE)
1200 19th St., N.W.
Suite 300
Washington, D.C. 20036
800-368-4404 (toll-free)

C/SEC inc. (Cesareans/Support Education and Concern)
22 Forest Road
Framingham, MA 01701
508-877-8266
Emotional support and information on cesarean births and vaginal birth after cesarean

National Organization of Mothers of Twins Clubs, Inc.
P.O. Box 23188
Albuquerque, NM 87192-1188
505-275-0955
Complimentary brochure and referral to nearest support group

Parents of Prematures
13613 NW 26th Place
Bellevue, WA 98005
Support for parents of premature babies

Parents Without Partners, Inc.
401 N. Michigan Ave.
Chicago, IL 60611-4267
800-637-7973 (toll-free)
Mutual support groups for parents and their children

POSTNATAL SUPPORT

American Association for Marriage and Family Therapy
1100 17th St., N.W.
Washington, D.C. 20006
202-452-0109
Provides lists of division presidents in your area

Childhelp U.S.A.
6463 Independence Ave.
Woodland Hills, CA 91367
800-4-A-CHILD (toll-free)
24-hour hotline for parents who think they might abuse their children or anyone reporting suspected child abuse

Compassionate Friends
P.O. Box 1347
Oak Brook, IL 60521
708-990-0010
Self-help group for those experiencing the death of a baby

Depression After Delivery
P.O. Box 1282
Morrisville, PA 19067
800-944-4773 (toll free)
Clearinghouse for emotional support through volunteer contacts throughout the US

International Childbirth Education Association
P. O. Box 20048
Minneapolis, MN 55420
612-854-8660
Listings of certified childbirth educators in your area

La Leche League International
P. O. Box 4079
Schaumburg, IL 60168-4079
708-519-7730
Breastfeeding information and support. (Check phone directory for local chapter or write to above address.)

Maternity Center Association
48 E. 92nd St.
New York, NY 10128
212-369 7300
Publications, videos on informed childbirth, especially 'natural childbirth'

National Association of Childbearing Centers
3123 Gottschall Road
Perkiomenville, PA 18074
Listing of freestanding birthing centers in your area; brochures (send $1 for shipping)

National Association of Parents and Professionals for Safe Alternatives in Childbirth
Route 1, Box 646
Marble Hill, M1 63764

National Down Syndrome Society
666 Broadway, 8th floor
New York, NY 10022-2317
800-221-4602 (toll-free)
Information and referrals

The March of Dimes
P.O. Box 2000
White Plains, NY 10602
Information and research on genetics, genetic counseling and birth defects

INFORMATION ON HEALTH, SAFETY AND FIRST AID

American Academy of Pediatrics
141 Northwest Point Blvd.
P.O. Box 927
Elk Grove Village. IL 60007
800-421-0589 (toll-free, IL only)
800-433-9016 (toll-free)
Information and referrals

American Red Cross
National Headquarters
17th and D Sts., N.W.
Washington, DC 20066
Publications on first aid and information regarding local first aid classes

Center for Science in the Public Interest
1875 Connecticut Ave., N.W.
Suite 300
Washington, D.C. 20099-5728
202-332-9110
Nutritional information and advocacy for a safe food supply

National Child Passenger Safety Association
Suite 300
1707 DeSales Street
Washington, D.C. 20036
202-429-0515
Answer questions on automobile safey

National Highway & Traffic Safety Administration
400 Seventh Street S.W.
Washington, D.C. 20590
800-424-9393 (auto safety hotline)
202-426-0123 (in Washington, D.C. only)
Information on infant and child safety seats

National Safety Council
444 N. Michigan Ave.
Chicago, IL 60611
312-527-4800
800-621-7619 (toll-free)
Information on safe toys and furniture, safety restraints, etc.

U.S. Consumer Product Safety Commission
1750 K St., N.W.
Washington, D.C. 20207
800-638-2772 (toll-free for information on recalls on children's toys and furniture; complaints about unsafe children's items)

i NDEX